Comparative Effectiveness Review
Number 142

Imaging Tests for the Staging of Colorectal Cancer

Prepared for:
Agency for Healthcare Research and Quality
U.S. Department of Health and Human Services
540 Gaither Road
Rockville, MD 20850
www.ahrq.gov

Contract No. 290-2012-00011-I

Prepared by:
ECRI Institute-Penn Medicine Evidence-based Practice Center
Plymouth Meeting, PA

Investigators:
Wendy Bruening, Ph.D.
Nancy Sullivan, B.A.
Emily Carter Paulson, M.D., M.S.C.E.
Hanna Zafar, M.D., M.H.S.
Matthew Mitchell, Ph.D.
Jonathan Treadwell, Ph.D.
Karen Schoelles, M.D., S.M., FACP

AHRQ Publication No. 14-EHC046-EF
September 2014

This report is based on research conducted by the ECRI Institute-Penn Medicine Evidence-based Practice Center (EPC) under contract to the Agency for Healthcare Research and Quality (AHRQ), Rockville, MD (Contract No. 290-2012-00011-I). The findings and conclusions in this document are those of the authors, who are responsible for its contents; the findings and conclusions do not necessarily represent the views of AHRQ. Therefore, no statement in this report should be construed as an official position of AHRQ or of the U.S. Department of Health and Human Services.

The information in this report is intended to help health care decisionmakers—patients and clinicians, health system leaders, and policymakers, among others—make well informed decisions and thereby improve the quality of health care services. This report is not intended to be a substitute for the application of clinical judgment. Anyone who makes decisions concerning the provision of clinical care should consider this report in the same way as any medical reference and in conjunction with all other pertinent information, i.e., in the context of available resources and circumstances presented by individual patients.

This report may be used, in whole or in part, as the basis for development of clinical practice guidelines and other quality enhancement tools, or as a basis for reimbursement and coverage policies. AHRQ or U.S. Department of Health and Human Services endorsement of such derivative products may not be stated or implied.

This report may periodically be assessed for the urgency to update. If an assessment is done, the resulting surveillance report describing the methodology and findings will be found on the Effective Health Care Program Web site at www.effectivehealthcare.ahrq.gov. Search on the title of the report.

This document is in the public domain and may be used and reprinted without special permission. Citation of the source is appreciated.

Persons using assistive technology may not be able to fully access information in this report. For assistance contact EffectiveHealthCare@ahrq.hhs.gov.

None of the investigators have any affiliations or financial involvement that conflicts with the material presented in this report.

Suggested citation: Bruening W, Sullivan N, Carter Paulson E, Zafar H, Mitchell M, Treadwell J, Schoelles K. Imaging Tests for the Staging of Colorectal Cancer. Comparative Effectiveness Review No. 142. (Prepared by the ECRI Institute-Penn Medicine Evidence-based Practice Center under Contract No. 290-2012-00011-I.) AHRQ Publication No. 14-EHC046-EF. Rockville, MD: Agency for Healthcare Research and Quality; September 2014. www.effectivehealthcare.ahrq.gov/reports/final.cfm.

Preface

The Agency for Healthcare Research and Quality (AHRQ), through its Evidence-based Practice Centers (EPCs), sponsors the development of systematic reviews to assist public- and private-sector organizations in their efforts to improve the quality of health care in the United States. These reviews provide comprehensive, science-based information on common, costly medical conditions, and new health care technologies and strategies.

Systematic reviews are the building blocks underlying evidence-based practice; they focus attention on the strength and limits of evidence from research studies about the effectiveness and safety of a clinical intervention. In the context of developing recommendations for practice, systematic reviews can help clarify whether assertions about the value of the intervention are based on strong evidence from clinical studies. For more information about AHRQ EPC systematic reviews, see www.effectivehealthcare.ahrq.gov/reference/purpose.cfm.

AHRQ expects that these systematic reviews will be helpful to health plans, providers, purchasers, government programs, and the health care system as a whole. Transparency and stakeholder input are essential to the Effective Health Care Program. Please visit the Web site (www.effectivehealthcare.ahrq.gov) to see draft research questions and reports or to join an email list to learn about new program products and opportunities for input.

We welcome comments on this systematic review. They may be sent by mail to the Task Order Officer named below at: Agency for Healthcare Research and Quality, 540 Gaither Road, Rockville, MD 20850, or by email to epc@ahrq.hhs.gov.

Richard G. Kronick, Ph.D.
Director
Agency for Healthcare Research and Quality

Yen-pin Chiang, Ph.D.
Acting Deputy Director
Center for Evidence and Practice Improvement
Agency for Healthcare Research and Quality

Stephanie Chang, M.D., M.P.H.
Director, EPC Program
Center for Evidence and Practice Improvement
Agency for Healthcare Research and Quality

Nahed El-Kassar, M.D., Ph.D.
Task Order Officer
Center for Evidence and Practice Improvement
Agency for Healthcare Research and Quality

Acknowledgments

The authors gratefully acknowledge the following individuals for their contributions to this project: Rebecca Rishar for conducting the searches and helping to screen abstracts, Gina Giradi for managing the project and recruiting the technical experts and reviewers, Dr. Craig Umscheid for recruiting clinical coauthors and technical reviewers, and for reviewing the final draft, and Lydia Dharia for spending endless hours formatting the report.

Key Informants

In designing the study questions, the EPC consulted several Key Informants who represent the end-users of research. The EPC sought the Key Informant input on the priority areas for research and synthesis. Key Informants are not involved in the analysis of the evidence or the writing of the report. Therefore, in the end, study questions, design, methodological approaches, and/or conclusions do not necessarily represent the views of individual Key Informants.

Key Informants must disclose any financial conflicts of interest greater than $10,000 and any other relevant business or professional conflicts of interest. Because of their role as end-users, individuals with potential conflicts may be retained. The TOO and the EPC work to balance, manage, or mitigate any conflicts of interest.

The list of Key Informants who participated in developing this report follows:

Ivy Ahmed, M.P.H.
Vice-President for Education & Outreach
Research in Training Institute, Cancer Support Community
Washington, DC

George J. Chang, M.D., M.S., FACS, FASCRS
Surgical Oncologist
MD Anderson Cancer Center
Houston, TX

George A. Fisher, Jr., M.D., Ph.D.
Gastrointestinal Oncologist
Stanford Cancer Center
Stanford, CAKoenraad J. Mortele, M.D.
Radiologist
Beth Israel Deaconess Medical Center
Boston, MA

Nancy Roach
Chair of Board of Directors, Fight Colorectal Cancer
Alexandria, VA

Max Rosen, M.D.
Chairman of Radiology
UMass Memorial Medical Center
Boston, MA

Roger Snow, M.D., M.P.H.
Deputy Medical Director,
Office of Clinical Affairs, Office of Medicaid
Massachusetts Department of Health and Human Services
Boston, MA

Wayne Wild, M.D., Ph.D.
Medical Director, Tufts Health Plan
Boston, MASandra L. Wong, M.D., M.S.
Associate Professor of Surgery
University of Michigan
Ann Arbor, MI

Technical Expert Panel

In designing the study questions and methodology at the outset of this report, the EPC consulted several technical and content experts. Broad expertise and perspectives were sought. Divergent and conflicted opinions are common and perceived as healthy scientific discourse that results in a thoughtful, relevant systematic review. Therefore, in the end, study questions, design, methodologic approaches, and/or conclusions do not necessarily represent the views of individual technical and content experts.

Technical Experts must disclose any financial conflicts of interest greater than $10,000 and any other relevant business or professional conflicts of interest. Because of their unique clinical or content expertise, individuals with potential conflicts may be retained. The TOO and the EPC work to balance, manage, or mitigate any potential conflicts of interest identified.

The list of Technical Experts who participated in developing this report follows:

Al B. Benson, III, M.D., FACP
Professor of Medicine, Division of Hematology/Oncology
Northwestern University Feinberg School of Medicine
Chicago, IL

Bruce J. Giantonio, M.D.
Associate Professor of Medicine
University of Pennsylvania Perelman School of Medicine
Philadelphia, PA

Najjia Mahmoud, M.D.
Chief, Division of Colon and Rectal Surgery
University of Pennsylvania Perelman School of Medicine
Philadelphia, PA

Max Rosen, M.D., M.P.H.
Chairman of Radiology
UMass Memorial Medical Center
Boston, MA

Mark A. Schattner, M.D., FACP, C.N.S.P.
Department of Gastroenterology and Preventive Oncology
Memorial Sloan-Kettering Cancer Center
New York, NY

Christopher Willett, M.D.
Chair, Radiation Oncology
Duke Cancer Center
Durham, NC

Sandra L. Wong, M.D., M.S.
Associate Professor of Surgery
University of Michigan
Ann Arbor, MI

Peer Reviewers

Prior to publication of the final evidence report, EPCs sought input from independent Peer Reviewers without financial conflicts of interest. However, the conclusions and synthesis of the scientific literature presented in this report do not necessarily represent the views of individual reviewers.

Peer Reviewers must disclose any financial conflicts of interest greater than $10,000 and any other relevant business or professional conflicts of interest. Because of their unique clinical or content expertise, individuals with potential nonfinancial conflicts may be retained. The TOO and the EPC work to balance, manage, or mitigate any potential nonfinancial conflicts of interest identified.

The list of Peer Reviewers follows:

Rongwei (Rochelle) Fu, Ph.D.
Associate Professor, Department of Public Health and Preventive Medicine
Oregon Health & Science University
Portland, OR

Benjamin Krevsky, M.D., M.P.H.
Professor of Medicine
Director of Gastrointestinal Endoscopy
Temple University School of Medicine
Philadelphia, PA

Srinivas Puli, M.D.
Gastroenterologist
OSF Medical Group
Peoria, IL

Larissa Temple, M.D., FACS, FRCS(C)
Colorectal Surgeon
Memorial Sloan-Kettering Cancer Center
New York, NY

Joel Tepper, M.D.
Department of Radiation Oncology
UNC/Lineberger Comprehensive Cancer Center
University of North Carolina School of Medicine
Chapel Hill, NC

Imaging Tests for the Staging of Colorectal Cancer

Structured Abstract

Objective. Colorectal cancer is both the third most common type of cancer and the third most common cause of cancer-related death for both men and women. Treatment options for colorectal cancer differ depending on the clinical stage of disease at diagnosis. Our objective was to synthesize the available evidence on the comparative effectiveness of imaging tests for staging colorectal cancer.

Data sources. We searched Embase®, MEDLINE®, PubMed, and the Cochrane Library from 1980 through November 2013 for published, English-language, full-length articles on using endoscopic rectal ultrasound (ERUS), computed tomography (CT), magnetic resonance imaging (MRI), and positron emission tomography (PET)/CT for staging colorectal cancer. The searches identified 4,683 citations; after dual screening against the inclusion criteria, 8 systematic reviews and 65 primary comparative studies were included.

Methods. We performed dual data abstraction from the included studies and constructed evidence tables. Where possible, we pooled the data using binomial-bivariate random-effects regression models (for diagnostic accuracy outcomes) or using random-effects meta-analysis (for under- and overstaging and under- and overtreatment outcomes). We rated the risk of bias of individual studies using internal validity instruments and graded the overall strength of evidence of conclusions using four domains (study limitations, consistency, precision, directness).

Results. Preoperative staging: For preoperative rectal cancer T (tumor) staging, ERUS is more accurate than CT; ERUS is less likely than CT to incorrectly stage (odds ratio [OR] = 0.36; 95% confidence interval [CI], 0.24 to 0.54), less likely to understage (OR = 0.63; 95% CI, 0.44 to 0.89), and less likely to overstage (OR = 0.47; 95% CI, 0.28 to 0.80), supported by evidence of low strength. For preoperative rectal cancer T staging, MRI and ERUS were similar in accuracy, supported by evidence of low strength. There was no statistical difference in accuracy between MRI and CT, but there were few patients in the available studies. For preoperative rectal cancer N (lymph node) staging, CT, MRI, and ERUS were similar in overall accuracy, but all three modalities had limited sensitivity. MRI was less likely to overstage preoperative rectal cancer N stage than CT (OR = 0.498; 95% CI, 0.308 to 0.806), supported by evidence of low strength. We identified only one study of preoperative T and N staging of colorectal cancer using CT versus PET/CT. Nine studies reported on preoperative colorectal M (metastasis) staging. MRI is more sensitive than CT for detecting colorectal liver metastases (OR = 1.3, 95% CI, 1.0 to 1.8), supported by evidence of moderate strength.

Restaging: There is no statistically significant difference in accuracy across MRI, CT, or ERUS for interim rectal T restaging, supported by evidence of low strength. The evidence was insufficient for drawing conclusions regarding other interim restaging outcomes for rectal or colorectal cancer following initial treatment.

Harms: While perforation, bleeding, and pain are potential complications of ERUS, most studies reporting complications mentioned only mild discomfort or minor bleeding. Rare but potential harms of MRI are associated with use of gadolinium-based contrast agents. Harms of CT include radiation exposure and adverse events from intravenous contrast agents.

Conclusions. ERUS is preferable to CT for preoperative rectal cancer T staging (based on evidence of low strength). Moderate-strength evidence suggests MRI is preferable to CT for detecting colorectal liver metastases. Low-strength evidence suggests that CT, MRI, and ERUS are comparable for rectal cancer N staging, where all have limited sensitivity, and for interim rectal cancer T restaging. Evidence was insufficient to allow any evidence-based conclusions about the use of PET/CT for colorectal cancer staging.

Contents

Executive Summary ES-1

Introduction 1
   Background 1
      Colorectal Cancer 1
      Staging 2
      Imaging Technologies 5
   Scope and Key Questions 9
      Scope of the Review 9
      Key Questions 13
      PICOTS 14
      Conceptual Framework 15
   Organization of This Report 17

Methods 18
   Topic Refinement and Review Protocol 18
   Literature Search Strategy 18
      Search Strategy 18
      Inclusion and Exclusion Criteria 18
      Study Selection 21
      Data Abstraction 21
   Individual Study Quality (Risk of Bias) Evaluation 21
   Data Analysis and Synthesis 22
   Strength of Evidence Grading 24
   Applicability 25
   Peer Review and Public Commentary 25

Results 26
   Introduction 26
   Results of Literature Searches 26
   Test Performance of Imaging Modalities for Pretreatment Staging 28
      Key Points 28
      Detailed Synthesis 34
   Comparative Test Performance of Imaging Modalities for Pretreatment Staging 37
      Key Points 37
      Detailed Synthesis 37
   Comparative and Additive Impact of Imaging Modalities on Stage Reclassification and Management 50
      Key Points 50
      Detailed Synthesis 50
   Comparative and Additive Impact of Imaging Modalities on Clinical Outcomes 51

Adverse Effects Associated With Imaging Techniques 51
    Key Points 51
    Detailed Synthesis 52
Factors Affecting Accuracy 55
    Key Points 55
    Detailed Synthesis 55
Conclusions for Key Question 1 56
Comparative Test Performance of Imaging Modalities for Restaging After Initial Treatment 58
    Key Points 59
    Systematic Reviews 59
    Detailed Synthesis 59
Comparative and Additive Impact of Imaging Modalities on Stage Reclassification and
Management 63
Comparative and Additive Impact of Imaging Modalities on Clinical Outcomes 63
Adverse Effects Associated With Imaging Techniques 63
Factors Affecting Accuracy 63
Conclusions for Key Question 2 63

Discussion 65
Key Findings and Strength of Evidence 65
Findings in Relationship to What Is Already Known 67
Applicability 69
Implications for Clinical and Policy Decisionmaking 69
Limitations of the Comparative Effectiveness Review Process 71
    Impact of Key Assumptions 71
    Decisions Related to Project Scope 72
Limitations of the Evidence Base 72
Research Gaps 73
Conclusions 74

References 75

Abbreviations and Acronyms 89

Glossary of Selected Terms 91

Tables

Table A. Accuracy of imaging tests as reported by recent systematic reviews
Table B. Summary results for primary preoperative rectal T staging
Table C. Summary results for primary preoperative rectal N staging
Table D. Pooled random-effects meta-analyses of preoperative colorectal M staging (per lesion basis)
Table E. Summary of major conclusions

Table 1.	Tumor-Node-Metastasis (TNM) definitions for colorectal cancer	3
Table 2.	Dukes system	4
Table 3.	Modified Astler-Coller system	4
Table 4.	Taxonomic and prognostic groups based on the AJCC, Dukes, and Modified Astler-Coller staging systems	4
Table 5.	Summary of existing guidelines for staging colorectal cancer	10
Table 6.	Included systematic reviews addressing accuracy of ERUS, MRI, CT, or PET/CT	29
Table 7.	Results from included systematic reviews for endoscopic rectal ultrasound	34
Table 8.	Results from included systematic reviews for computed tomography	35
Table 9.	Results from included systematic reviews for MRI	36
Table 10.	Results from included systematic reviews of PET/CT	36
Table 11.	Results from included primary studies for PET/CT	37
Table 12.	Preoperative rectal T staging	38
Table 13.	Summary results for primary preoperative rectal T staging	40
Table 14.	Preoperative rectal nodal staging	44
Table 15.	Summary results for rectal N staging	46
Table 16.	Rectal N staging: differences between studies in various factors	46
Table 17.	Preoperative colorectal M staging	49
Table 18.	Pooled random-effects analyses for preoperative colorectal M staging (per lesion basis)	49
Table 19.	Accuracy of imaging tests as reported by recent systematic reviews	57
Table 20.	Results from included systematic review of interim restaging	59
Table 21.	Interim rectal T restaging	60
Table 22.	Interim rectal N restaging	60
Table 23.	Details of studies of interim rectal N restaging	61
Table 24.	Interim colorectal M restaging	62
Table 25.	Accuracy of imaging tests in isolation as reported by recent systematic reviews	65
Table 26.	Summary of major conclusions	66

Figures

Figure 1. Analytical framework of colorectal cancer staging review 16
Figure 2. Study flow diagram 27
Figure 3. MRI versus ERUS accuracy for rectal T staging 41
Figure 4. CT versus ERUS: risk of rectal T overstaging 42
Figure 5. CT versus ERUS: risk of rectal T understaging 42
Figure 6. MRI versus CT rectal T accuracy 43

Appendixes

Appendix A. Search Strategy
Appendix B. Excluded Studies
Appendix C. Evidence Tables
Appendix D. Analyses and Risk of Bias Assessments

Executive Summary

Background

Colorectal Cancer

In the United States each year colon cancer is diagnosed in approximately 100,000 people and rectal cancer is diagnosed in another 50,000.[1] Colorectal cancer usually affects older adults, with 90 percent of cases diagnosed in individuals 50 years of age and older.[2] Colorectal cancer is often fatal, with approximately 50,000 deaths attributed to it each year in the United States.[1] As such, it is both the third most common type of cancer and the third most common cause of cancer-related death for both men and women. Health care costs associated with care of these cancers is high, second only to breast cancer.[3,4]

Colorectal cancers may be diagnosed during screening of asymptomatic individuals or after a person has developed symptoms. Colon cancer symptoms include abdominal discomfort, change in bowel habits, anemia, and weight loss. Rectal cancer symptoms include bleeding, diarrhea, and pain. The U.S. Preventive Services Task Force currently recommends screening for colorectal cancer in asymptomatic normal-risk individuals using fecal occult blood testing, sigmoidoscopy, or colonoscopy, beginning at age 50 years and continuing until age 75 years.[5] Diagnosis is usually established through histopathologic examination of tissue samples (most often obtained through biopsies performed during colonoscopy).

Staging

Once the diagnosis has been established, patients with colorectal cancer undergo testing to establish the extent of disease spread, known as clinical staging. Staging is used primarily to determine appropriate initial treatment strategies. For colorectal cancer, the American Joint Committee on Cancer (AJCC) endorses the widely accepted "TNM" staging system. The AJCC system aims to characterize the anatomic extent of colorectal cancer based on three tumor characteristics: the extent of tumor infiltration into the bowel wall (tumor stage, designated as "T"), the extent of local or regional lymph node spread (nodal stage, designated as "N"), and the presence of distant metastatic lesions (metastatic spread, designated as "M").

Treatment options for colorectal cancer differ depending on the clinical stage of disease at diagnosis. For example, tumors confined to the rectal wall can be treated primarily by upfront surgical resection, but tumors that have penetrated the bowel wall usually require preoperative chemotherapy and radiation (neoadjuvant therapy) prior to definitive surgical resection. Clinical stage is not the only determinant of treatment options; patient comorbidities and preferences and clinician and institution preferences are also used in decisionmaking. However, stage is the key determinant of the management strategy. Staging is also used to inform patient prognosis and identify patients at higher risk of relapse or cancer-related mortality.

Clinical staging is performed at two distinct timepoints in the management of colorectal cancer. The first is immediately after diagnosis, before any treatment has been given. Imaging and clinical examination are used to assign a clinical stage, which is used to make decisions about primary treatment and management. The second timepoint (interim restaging) applies only to patients who, on the basis of their primary staging, were treated with neoadjuvant chemotherapy or radiotherapy instead of by immediate surgery. Chemotherapy/radiotherapy affects the metabolism and structure of the tissues such that some forms of imaging may be less accurate for restaging than in the pretreatment setting. Also, the role of imaging at each of these two timepoints is very different, and for these reasons they are addressed in separate Key Questions in this review.

Objectives of This Review

The primary objective of this review is to synthesize the available information on the comparative accuracy and effectiveness of imaging for staging of colorectal cancer. The availability of this information will assist clinicians in selecting protocols for staging, may reduce variability across treatment centers in staging protocols, and may improve patient outcomes. A secondary objective is to identify gaps in the evidence base to inform future research needs.

Key Questions and Scope

Key Questions

The Key Questions are listed below.

Key Question 1. What is the comparative effectiveness of imaging techniques for pretreatment cancer staging in patients with primary and recurrent colorectal cancer?

a. What is the test performance of the imaging techniques used (singly, in combination, or in a specific sequence) to stage colorectal cancer compared with a reference standard?
b. What is the impact of alternative imaging techniques on intermediate outcomes, including stage reclassification and changes in therapeutic management?
c. What is the impact of alternative imaging techniques on clinical outcomes?
d. What are the adverse effects or harms associated with using imaging techniques, including harms of test-directed management?
e. How is the comparative effectiveness of imaging techniques modified by the following factors:
    i. Patient-level characteristics (e.g., age, sex, body mass index)?
    ii. Disease characteristics (e.g., tumor grade)?
    iii. Imaging technique or protocol characteristics (e.g., use of different tracers or contrast agents, radiation dose of the imaging modality, slice thickness, timing of contrast)?

Key Question 2. What is the comparative effectiveness of imaging techniques for restaging cancer in patients with primary and recurrent colorectal cancer after initial treatment?

a. What is the test performance of the imaging techniques used (singly, in combination, or in a specific sequence) to restage colorectal cancer compared with a reference standard?
b. What is the impact of alternative imaging techniques on intermediate outcomes, including stage reclassification and changes in therapeutic management?
c. What is the impact of alternative imaging techniques on clinical outcomes?
d. What are the adverse effects or harms associated with using imaging techniques, including harms of test-directed management?

e. How is the comparative effectiveness of imaging techniques modified by the following factors:
    i. Patient-level characteristics (e.g., age, sex, body mass index)?
    ii. Disease characteristics (e.g., tumor grade)?
    iii. Imaging technique or protocol characteristics (e.g., use of different tracers or contrast agents, radiation dose of the imaging modality, slice thickness, timing of contrast)?

Scope

An analytic framework showing the populations, interventions, comparators, outcomes, timing, and setting (PICOTS) in diagram form is shown in Figure 1 of the full report.

Populations:
- Adult patients with an established diagnosis of primary colorectal cancer
- Adult patients with an established diagnosis of recurrent colorectal cancer

Interventions:
Noninvasive imaging using the following tests (alone or in combination) for assessing the stage of colorectal cancer:
- Endoscopic rectal ultrasound (ERUS)
- Computed tomography (CT)
- Magnetic resonance imaging (MRI)
- Positron emission tomography combined with computed tomography (PET/CT)

Reference Standards To Assess Test Performance:
- Histopathologic examination of tissue
- Intraoperative findings
- Clinical followup

Comparators:
- Any direct comparisons of the imaging tests of interest
- Any direct comparisons of variations of any of the imaging tests of interest (e.g., diffusion-weighted MRI vs. T2-weighted MRI)

Outcomes:
- Test performance outcomes
    - Test performance (sensitivity, specificity, accuracy, understaging, overstaging)
- Intermediate outcomes
    - Stage reclassification
    - Changes in therapeutic management
- Clinical outcomes
    - Overall mortality
    - Colorectal cancer–specific mortality
    - Quality of life and anxiety
    - Need for additional staging tests, including invasive procedures
    - Need for additional treatment, including surgery, radiotherapy, or chemotherapy
    - Resource use related to testing and treatment
- Adverse effects and harms

- o Harms of testing per se (e.g., radiation exposure)
- o Harms from test-directed treatments (e.g., overtreatment, undertreatment)

Timing:
- Primary staging
- Interim restaging

Setting:
All settings were considered.

Methods

Search Strategy

Medical librarians in the Evidence-based Practice Center (EPC) Information Center performed literature searches following established systematic review protocols. We searched the following databases from 1980 through November 2013 using controlled vocabulary and text words: Embase®, MEDLINE®, PubMed, and the Cochrane Library. The full search strategy is shown in Appendix A of the full report.

Literature screening was performed in duplicate using the database DistillerSR (Evidence Partners, Ottawa, Canada). Initially, we screened literature search results in duplicate (two screeners) for relevancy. We screened relevant abstracts again, in duplicate, against the inclusion and exclusion criteria. Studies that appeared to meet the inclusion criteria were retrieved in full, and we screened them again, in duplicate, against the inclusion and exclusion criteria. All disagreements were resolved by consensus discussion among the two original screeners and, if necessary, an additional third screener.

Study Selection

Criteria for Inclusion and Exclusion of Studies in the Review

The inclusion/exclusion criteria were—

1. *Publication type.* The article must have been published as a full-length, English-language, peer-reviewed study. Abstracts and meeting presentations were excluded.
2. *Single test performance.* For questions about the performance of a single imaging test against a reference standard, we used a two-stage inclusion process. We first included only recent (2009 or later) high-quality systematic reviews. We included primary studies (1980 or later) only if the evidence from systematic reviews was insufficient to support an estimate of test performance for a particular imaging test.
3. *Comparative test performance.* For questions about comparative test performance, we considered studies of any design—randomized, cross-sectional, case-control, or cohort—for inclusion. Both retrospective and prospective studies were considered for inclusion, but retrospective studies must have used consecutive/all enrollment or enrollment of a random sample of participants. Studies must have directly compared the tests with each other and with a reference standard; all tests being compared must have been evaluated by the same reference standard.
4. *Stage reclassification or clinical decision impact.* For questions about stage reclassification or impact on clinician decisionmaking, cross-sectional, cohort, or

prospective comparative (randomized or nonrandomized) studies were considered for inclusion.

5. *Clinical outcomes.* For questions about the impact of testing on patient-oriented clinical outcomes, we considered comparative studies (randomized or nonrandomized, prospective or retrospective) for inclusion.
6. *Harms.* The adverse events and harms reported by any studies included to address any of the other questions were used to address questions about harms and adverse events. In addition, we searched specifically for reports of harms and adverse events associated with the use of each specific imaging modality, such as radiation exposure and reactions to contrast agents. Any study design, including modeling, was acceptable for inclusion for questions about harms.
7. *Type of patient.* For inclusion, the study must have reported data obtained from groups in which at least 85 percent of patients were from one of the four patient populations of interest: (1) patients with newly diagnosed colorectal cancer underdoing primary staging, (2) patients with newly diagnosed colorectal cancer undergoing interim restaging, (3) patients with newly diagnosed recurrent colorectal cancer undergoing primary staging, and (4) patients with newly diagnosed recurrent colorectal cancer undergoing interim restaging.
8. *Adults.* Only studies of adult patients (18 years of age and older) were considered for inclusion.
9. *Obsolete technology.* The Technical Expert Panel was consulted a priori about which imaging technologies and variants of imaging technologies are obsolete and not relevant to clinical practice, and these were excluded. Likewise, experimental technologies and prototypes were excluded. The imaging technologies that were determined, after discussion and consensus, to be obsolete for staging colorectal cancer are transabdominal ultrasound, MRI using endorectal coils, nonmultidetector CT, CT arterial portography, CT angiography, CT colonography, and stand-alone PET. The Technical Expert Panel indicated that PET/MRI and PET fused with CT colonography are considered to be experimental. MRI using ultrasmall paramagnetic iron oxide is also considered experimental
10. *Number of patients.* We included data from timepoints and outcomes reported from groups with at least 10 patients with the condition of interest who represented at least 50 percent of the patients originally enrolled in the study. We included case series, but not individual case reports, in the search for harms.

Criteria for Key Questions on Harms

While we utilized data from studies meeting the inclusion criteria above for questions about harms, we supplemented this information with information from narrative reviews and other sources, such as U.S. Food and Drug Administration (FDA) alerts. Additionally, we systematically searched for information on harms related to the various imaging modalities of interest (regardless of condition or disease state). Our search strategy is shown in Appendix A.

Our inclusion criteria for the supplemental harms searches were—

1. Articles must have been published in English.
2. Articles must have specifically focused on adverse events from ERUS, CT, MRI, or PET/CT, but any patient population or disease was acceptable.

3. Clinical studies had to be published in 2008 or later (to include the most current literature only).
4. Narrative reviews had to be published in 2012 or later.

Data Abstraction

We abstracted data using the database DistillerSR (Evidence Partners Incorporated, Ottawa, Canada). Data abstraction forms were constructed in Distiller, and we extracted the data into these forms. Duplicate abstraction was used to ensure accuracy.

Elements that were abstracted include general study characteristics, patient characteristics, details of the imaging methodology, risk-of-bias items, and outcome data.

Individual Study Quality (Risk-of-Bias) Evaluation

We used internal validity rating instruments to evaluate the risk of bias of each individual study. The instruments are shown in Appendix D. Studies were rated as low, medium, or high risk of bias. The ratings were defined by selecting critical questions from a rating scale that must be answered "yes." We selected the critical questions for these ratings for the review after discussions with the Technical Expert Panel.

As suggested by the "Methods Guide for Effectiveness and Comparative Effectiveness Reviews" (Methods Guide), systematic reviews used to address Key Questions 1a and 2a were evaluated for risk of bias with a modified AMSTAR instrument,[6] which is shown in Appendix C. Systematic reviews were rated as either high quality or not. The rating was defined by selecting critical questions from the rating scale that must be answered "yes." The critical questions for these ratings for the review were selected after discussions with the Technical Expert Panel. Only high-quality systematic reviews were included to address Key Questions 1a and 2a.

Strength-of-Evidence Grading

We used a formal grading system that conforms with the Methods Guide recommendations on grading the strength of evidence.[7-9]

The overall strength of evidence supporting each major conclusion was graded as high, moderate, low, or insufficient. The grade was developed by considering four important domains: study limitations (based on the risk of bias of the individual studies addressing a question), consistency of the findings, precision of the results, and directness of the evidence. The grades are defined as follows:

- *High.* We are very confident that the estimate of effect lies close to the true effect for this outcome. The body of evidence has few or no deficiencies. We believe that the findings are stable—that is, another study would not change the conclusions.
- *Moderate.* We are moderately confident that the estimate of effect lies close to the true effect for this outcome. The body of evidence has some deficiencies. We believe that the findings are likely to be stable, but some doubt remains.
- *Low.* We have limited confidence that the estimate of effect lies close to the true effect for this outcome. The body of evidence has major or numerous deficiencies (or both). We believe that additional evidence is needed before concluding either that the findings are stable or that the estimate of effect is close to the true effect.

- *Insufficient.* We have no evidence, we are unable to estimate an effect, or we have no confidence in the estimate of effect for this outcome. No evidence is available or the body of evidence has unacceptable deficiencies, precluding reaching a conclusion.

We did not grade the strength of evidence from published systematic reviews on the accuracy of individual imaging tests.

Applicability

The applicability of the evidence involves four key aspects: patients, tests/interventions, comparisons, and settings. After discussions with the Technical Expert Panel, we concluded that age and sex of patients are unlikely to affect staging accuracy, but other patient characteristics, such as race, obesity, genetic syndromes predisposing to colorectal cancer, and enrollment of populations with high rates of comorbid conditions, could affect the applicability of study findings, particularly with regard to patient-oriented outcomes. To improve the applicability of the findings regarding specific tests and comparisons, we excluded obsolete and experimental imaging tests.

Data Analysis and Synthesis

For questions addressing individual test performance (accuracy), we used evidence from earlier systematic reviews. As recommended by the Methods Guide, we summarized all relevant high-quality reviews.[6] (See above for a definition of high-quality systematic reviews.)

For comparative questions, we synthesized the evidence from the primary studies themselves. We performed meta-analysis wherever appropriate and possible. Decisions about whether meta-analysis was appropriate were based on the judged clinical homogeneity of the different study populations, imaging and treatment protocols, and outcomes. When meta-analysis was not possible (because of limitations of reported data) or was judged to be inappropriate, the data were synthesized using a descriptive approach.

Consistency of the evidence was assessed by considering study populations, imaging and treatment protocols, study designs, and outcomes, in addition to statistical heterogeneity. We rated the consistency of conclusions supported by random-effects meta-analyses with the statistic I^2. For qualitative comparisons, we rated conclusions as consistent if the effect sizes were all in the same direction.

For studies of clinical outcomes and analyses of accuracy, overstaging, and understaging, we computed effect sizes (odds ratios [ORs] of making errors) and measures of variance using standard methods and performed DerSimonian and Laird random-effects meta-analyses using Comprehensive Meta-Analysis (CMA) software (Biostat, Inc., Englewood, NJ). Because the same patients underwent both tests being compared and studies did not report the correlations among tests, we assumed a correlation of 0.5 and performed sensitivity analyses using correlations of 0.1 and 0.9.

To analyze diagnostic test characteristics, the data must first be dichotomized. For N staging, dichotomization is straightforward: the lymph nodes are affected (N1, N2) or are not affected (N0). For M staging, the situation is similar. For T staging, dichotomization is not as straightforward; however, after considering the clinical situation, a clinically relevant dichotomization is apparent: groups T1/T2 together and T3/T4 together. This dichotomization is clinically relevant because treatment of T1/T2 colorectal cancer is similar, treatment of T3/T4 is similar, and treatment of T1/T2 versus T3/T4 is very different. After dichotomization, for studies of test performance (sensitivity, specificity), we meta-analyzed the data reported by the studies using a binomial-bivariate random-effects regression model, as described by Harbord et al.[10] All such analyses were computed by the STATA 13.0 statistical software package using the metandi command.[11] In cases in which a bivariate binomial regression model could not be fit to the available data, we meta-analyzed the diagnostic data using a random-effects model and the software package Meta-Disc (freeware developed by the Unit of Clinical Biostatistics, Ramón y Cajal Hospital, Madrid, Spain).[12]

Wherever possible, we performed calculations of standard diagnostic test characteristics (sensitivity, specificity) and also calculations of accuracy, understaging, and overstaging. If the two different approaches to analysis produced different conclusions about which test is to be preferred for that situation, the data were categorized as inconsistent/heterogeneous.

We explored possible causes of heterogeneity with subgroup analysis. Covariates included population descriptors, tumor site and type, country and setting of care, variations in imaging technology, and publication date.

Peer Review and Publication

Peer reviewers were invited to provide written comments on the draft report based on their clinical, content, or methodologic expertise. The EPC considered peer-review comments on the preliminary draft of the report in preparation of the final report. The dispositions of the peer-review comments are documented and will be published 3 months after publication of the report.

Results

Evidence Base

The literature searches identified 4,683 citations. After review of the abstracts of these articles in duplicate, 4,473 were excluded. The most common reason for exclusion was lack of relevancy to the questions. Some of the excluded narrative reviews and patterns-of-care articles were used to inform the background section and the patterns-of-care discussion in the final chapter of the full report. In all, 210 articles were retrieved in full: 31 were screened against the systematic review inclusion criteria, and 179 were screened against the clinical study inclusion criteria. See the Methods section for lists of the inclusion criteria. After screening the articles in duplicate, we included 8 systematic reviews and 65 primary clinical studies. See Appendix B for a list of the excluded studies.

Key Question 1. What is the comparative effectiveness of imaging techniques for pretreatment cancer staging in patients with primary and recurrent colorectal cancer?

Key Question 1a. What is the test performance of the imaging techniques used (singly, in combination, or in a specific sequence) to stage colorectal cancer compared with a reference standard?

Seven recent (2009 or later) high-quality systematic reviews and 38 primary comparative studies met the inclusion criteria for this question. We compiled data from the recent high-quality systematic reviews to estimate the accuracy of each individual imaging modality in isolation. These data are summarized in Table A. One of the seven systematic reviews evaluated only a particular type of ERUS (miniprobes), so we did not include information from it in Table A due to concerns about generalizability. Because there were insufficient data on PET/CT from systematic reviews, we examined the studies of PET/CT addressing the comparative questions in this report to obtain an estimate of accuracy.

Table A. Accuracy of imaging tests as reported by recent systematic reviews

Staging	ERUS	CT	MRI	PET/CT
Rectal T	For identifying T1: Sensitivity: 87.8% (85.3% to 90.0%) Specificity: 98.3% (97.8% to 98.7%) For identifying T2: Sensitivity: 80.5% (77.9% to 82.9%) Specificity: 95.6% (94.9% to 96.3%) For identifying T3: Sensitivity: 96.4% (95.4% to 97.2%) Specificity: 90.6% (89.5% to 91.7%) For identifying T4: Sensitivity: 95.4% (92.4% to 97.5%) Specificity: 98.3% (97.8% to 98.7%)	For distinguishing T1/T2 from T3/T4: Sensitivity: 86% (78% to 92%) Specificity: 78% (71% to 84%)	For distinguishing T1/T2 from T3/T4: Sensitivity: 87% (81% to 92%) Specificity: 75% (68% to 80%) For identifying affected CRM: Sensitivity: 77% (57% to 90%) Specificity: 94% (88% to 97%)	Not reported
Rectal N	For identifying affected nodes: Sensitivity: 73.2% (70.6% to 75.6%) Specificity: 75.8% (73.5% to 78.0%)	For identifying affected nodes: Sensitivity: 70% (59% to 80%) Specificity: 78% (66% to 86%)	For identifying affected nodes: Sensitivity: 77% (69% to 84%) Specificity: 71% (59% to 81%)	For identifying affected nodes: Sensitivity: 61% Specificity: 83%
Colorectal T	Not reported	Not reported	Not reported	Accuracy: 95%
Colorectal N	Not reported	Not reported	Not reported	For identifying affected nodes: Sensitivity: 34.3% Specificity: 100%
Colorectal M	Not indicated	For identifying liver metastases: Sensitivity: 83.6%	For identifying liver metastases: Sensitivity: 88.2%	For identifying liver metastases: Sensitivity: 72.0% to 97.9%

Note: The 95% confidence intervals are shown in parentheses.
CRM = circumferential resection margin; CT = computed tomography; ERUS = endorectal ultrasound; M = metastases stage; MRI = magnetic resonance imaging; N = nodal stage; PET/CT = positron emission tomography/computed tomography; T = tumor stage.

To determine the comparative effectiveness of the different modalities, we examined studies that directly compared modalities with each other and verified the results with a reference standard (usually histopathology/intraoperative findings).

We identified 23 studies of preoperative rectal T staging. Six studies compared MRI with ERUS, 13 compared CT with ERUS, 3 compared MRI with CT, and 1 study compared CT, MRI, and ERUS. If possible, we fit a binomial-bivariate normal regression model to diagnostics accuracy data, and we performed random-effects meta-analyses on the measures of accuracy, overstaging, and understaging. The results of our calculations are shown in Table B.

Table B. Summary results for primary preoperative rectal T staging

Test Characteristics	MRI vs. ERUS	ERUS vs. CT	MRI vs. CT
Sensitivity (95% CI) of T1/T2 vs. T3/T4	MRI: 88.9% (79.0% to 94.4%) ERUS: 88.0% (80.0% to 93.1%)	Not calculated due to insufficient data reported	Not calculated
Specificity (95% CI) of T1/T2 vs. T3/T4	MRI: 85.3% (70.6% to 93.4%) ERUS: 85.6% (65.8% to 94.9%)	Not calculated due to insufficient data reported	Not calculated
Accuracy: OR of getting an incorrect result (95% CI)[a]	1.24 (0.835 to 1.84)	0.359 (0.238 to 0.541)	0.317 (0.056 to 1.784)[b]
Understaging OR (95% CI)[a]	1.571 (0.605 to 4.083)	0.626 (0.438 to 0.894)	0.317 (0.027 to 3.646)[b]
Overstaging OR (95% CI)[a]	1.05 (0.518 to 2.16)	0.472 (0.28 to 0.798)	0.317 (0.028 to 3.653)[b]
Favors	No statistically significant difference	ERUS	No statistically significant difference

[a]OR < 1 indicates a lower risk of error in the first imaging modality listed in the column header; OR > 1 indicates a higher risk of error in the first imaging modality listed in the column header.
[b]Study with 0.15T magnet excluded from analyses.

CI = confidence interval; CT = computed tomography; ERUS = endorectal ultrasound; MRI = magnetic resonance imaging; OR = odds ratio; T = tumor stage.

We identified 19 studies that reported data on rectal N staging. One study compared MRI with PET/CT, five compared MRI with ERUS, nine compared CT with ERUS, and four compared MRI with CT. If possible, we fit a binomial-bivariate normal regression model to diagnostics accuracy data, and we performed random-effects meta-analyses on the measures of accuracy, overstaging, and understaging. The results of our calculations are shown in Table C. The MRI versus PET/CT comparison (single study) was not statistically significant (0.467; confidence interval [CI], 0.193 to 1.130).

Table C. Summary results for primary preoperative rectal N staging

Test Characteristics	MRI vs. ERUS	CT vs. ERUS	MRI vs. CT
Sensitivity (95% CI)	MRI: 49.5% (36.0% to 63.1%) ERUS: 53.0% (39.7% to 65.5%)	CT: 39.6% (28.1% to 52.4%) ERUS: 49.1% (34.9% to 63.5%)	Not calculated
Specificity (95% CI)	MRI: 69.7% (51.9% to 83.0%) ERUS: 73.7% (43.6% to 91.0%)	CT: 93.2% (58.8% to 99.2%) ERUS: 71.7% (56.2% to 83.4%)	Not calculated
Accuracy: OR of getting an incorrect result (95% CI)[a]	0.882 (0.542 to 1.408)	1.13 (0.85 to 1.503)	1.316 (0.709 to 2.443)
Understaging OR (95% CI)[a]	0.972 (0.563 to 1.679)	1.453 (0.854 to 2.473)	1.743 (1.028 to 2.957); not robust in sensitivity analysis
Overstaging OR (95% CI)[a]	0.752 (0.457 to 1.237)	1.015 (0.571 to 1.801)	0.498 (0.308 to 0.806)
Favors	No statistically significant difference	No statistically significant difference	MRI favored for avoiding overstaging

[a]OR < 1 indicates a lower risk of error in the first imaging modality listed in the column header; OR > 1 indicates a higher risk of error in the first imaging modality listed in the column header.

CI = confidence interval; CT = computed tomography; ERUS = endorectal ultrasound; MRI = magnetic resonance imaging; N = nodal stage; OR = odds ratio.

We identified nine studies of preoperative colorectal M staging. Four compared PET/CT with CT, and five compared MRI with CT. Where possible, we fit a binomial-bivariate normal regression model to diagnostics accuracy data, and we performed random-effects meta-analyses on the measures of accuracy, overstaging, and understaging. The results of our calculations are shown in Table D. The statistical heterogeneity of the PET/CT data makes it difficult to draw any conclusions about the comparison with CT, and in fact, the conclusions drawn by the individual study authors ranged from no difference, to superiority of CT, to superiority of PET/CT for this purpose.

Table D. Pooled random-effects meta-analyses of preoperative colorectal M staging (per lesion basis)

Measure	MRI vs. CT	PET/CT vs. CT
Sensitivity	Not calculated	CT: 83.6% (95% CI, 78.1% to 88.2%) PET/CT: 60.4% (95% CI, 53.7% to 66.9%)
Summary OR for lesion detection[a]	1.334 (95% CI, 1.012 to 1.761)	Not calculated
I^2	12.4%	CT: 0.0% PET/CT: 95.1%
Favors	MRI	Insufficient evidence

[a] OR > 1 indicates a higher likelihood of detecting metastatic lesions by the first imaging modality listed in the column header.
CI = confidence interval; CT = computed tomography; M = metastases stage; MRI = magnetic resonance imaging; OR = odds ratio; PET/CT = positron emission tomography/computed tomography.

We identified only one study each of preoperative circumferential resection margin (CRM) status (MRI vs. CT) and colorectal T staging (CT vs. PET/CT).

We did not identify any studies of staging enrolling only patients who had colon cancer (i.e., results not combined with those for patients who had rectal cancer) that met the inclusion criteria.

Key Question 1b. What is the impact of alternative imaging techniques on intermediate outcomes, including stage reclassification and changes in therapeutic management?

We identified seven primary comparative studies that addressed this question.

Two studies reported on patient management based on MRI or ERUS for preoperative rectal staging. Both studies used a similar design. For each patient, the investigators devised a theoretical treatment strategy based solely on MRI information; they devised another theoretical treatment strategy based solely on ERUS information; and then they used a third strategy based on clinical information, MRI, and ERUS data to actually treat the patient. The histopathology after surgery was used to define the "correct" treatment strategy that should have been used. We pooled the results from both studies in a random-effects meta-analysis. We analyzed the outcomes "correct treatment," "undertreatment," and "overtreatment." All three analyses favored MRI as the more accurate modality for treatment planning, but none reached statistical significance.

Two studies that met the inclusion criteria reported the impact of adding PET/CT results to CT results for preoperative staging of colorectal cancer. One study did not measure whether the changes were appropriate. The other study reported that adding PET/CT to CT results changed management for 17.5 percent of patients, but after treatment, surgery, and followup, results indicated that only half of the changed treatment plans were the appropriate choice.

Two studies that met the inclusion criteria reported the impact of adding ERUS information to CT results, and one study reported the impact of adding PET/CT to MRI and CT for preoperative staging of rectal cancer. However, none of these studies verified whether the changes were appropriate.

Key Question 1c. What is the impact of alternative imaging techniques on clinical outcomes?

We did not identify any studies that addressed this question.

Key Question 1d. What are the adverse effects or harms associated with using imaging techniques, including harms of test-directed management?

To address this question, we abstracted data about harms reported by the included studies to address the questions on comparative accuracy in this report. We supplemented this information with information from narrative reviews and other sources (e.g., FDA alerts). Additionally, we systematically searched for information on harms related to the various imaging modalities of interest (regardless of condition or disease state). Our search strategy is shown in Appendix A. Our supplemental searches identified 1,961 abstracts; after review of these abstracts, we selected 66 articles to review in full text, of which 32 were selected for inclusion.

Ultrasound is generally considered to be extremely safe. For rectal imaging, an additional consideration is the fact that an endorectal probe is used; the probe is inserted into the rectum. Possible complications include perforation, bleeding, and pain. The majority of included studies of ERUS did not report any complications; whether this means that none occurred is unclear. Six studies reported adverse events such as pain and minor rectal bleeding. Four studies reported failure to complete the procedure because of stenosis or strictures. No studies reported any cases of perforation.

The supplemental harms searches identified one review of endoscopic ultrasound–related adverse events that included information on complications of ERUS. The authors reported that a large multicenter prospective German registry of endoscopic ultrasound procedures reported one perforation related to ERUS.

None of the included studies reported any adverse events related to CT or PET/CT. The supplemental harms searches identified reports of reactions to intravenous contrast agents. CT and PET/CT scans also expose the body to x rays. A typical abdominal CT scan exposes the body to approximately 10 mSv of radiation, and a typical PET/CT scan exposes the body to 18 mSv.

Only two of the included studies reported adverse events due to MRI, and both were reports of patients refusing the procedure because of severe claustrophobia. The supplemental harms searches identified the possibility of adverse events due to intravenous contrast agents, such as allergic reactions and nephrogenic systemic fibrosis, a scleroderma-like fibrosing condition that occurs in patients with renal failure and can be fatal. Labeling for gadolinium-based contrast agents now includes a warning regarding the risk of nephrogenic systemic fibrosis in patients with severe kidney insufficiency, patients just before or just after liver transplantation, or individuals with chronic liver disease.

Key Question 1e. How is the comparative effectiveness of imaging techniques modified by the following factors:

i. Patient-level characteristics (e.g., age, sex, body mass index)?
ii. Disease characteristics (e.g., tumor grade)?
iii. Imaging technique or protocol characteristics (e.g., use of different tracers or contrast agents, radiation dose of the imaging modality, slice thickness, timing of contrast)?

We identified 16 primary comparative studies that addressed this question.

Nine studies reported factors affecting MRI's accuracy for colorectal staging. Most of these studies reported on different factors; however, three studies reported that contrast enhancement did not improve MRI's accuracy for rectal T and N staging.

Five studies reported factors affecting the accuracy of ERUS for colorectal staging, and three studies reported factors affecting CT's accuracy for colorectal staging, but they reported on different factors, making it difficult to determine how any specific factors impact accuracy.

Conclusions for Key Question 1

For rectal T staging, ERUS and MRI appear to not be statistically significantly different in accuracy, and ERUS is more accurate than CT. There were no statistically significant differences in accuracy between MRI and CT for rectal T staging. The evidence was insufficient for drawing conclusions about the accuracy of PET/CT compared with either MRI or CT for rectal T staging.

For rectal N staging, ERUS, MRI, and CT are not significantly different in accuracy, but they all have low sensitivity for detecting affected lymph nodes. MRI is less likely to overstage and CT may be less likely to understage N status (although the latter conclusion was not robust in sensitivity analyses). The evidence was insufficient for drawing conclusions about the accuracy of PET/CT compared with either MRI or CT for rectal N staging.

For detecting colorectal liver metastases, MRI is superior to CT. The evidence was insufficient for drawing conclusions about the accuracy of PET/CT compared with either MRI or CT for colorectal M staging.

The evidence base is characterized by a lack of studies reporting patient-oriented outcomes. Seven studies reported on the impact of imaging on patient management, but only three of these studies confirmed whether the change in management was appropriate. In general, the included studies reported only on diagnostic accuracy. They were all rated as either low or moderate risk of bias.

A systematic review published in 2005 (thus not included to address the Key Questions) concluded that "the performance of EUS [endoscopic ultrasound] in staging rectal cancer may be overestimated in the literature due to publication bias."[13] The review included 41 studies published between 1985 and 2003. The author, Harewood, performed visual analyses of funnel plots and other diagrams, demonstrating that it appeared that few smaller studies found lower accuracy rates for ERUS and that the reported accuracy appeared to be declining over time. Studies published in the surgical literature reported higher accuracies than studies published in other types of journals.[13]

Puli et al. also analyzed the reported accuracy of ERUS over time and found that the reported accuracy had declined significantly from the 1980s through 2000 and had stabilized or only declined slightly since then.[14] Puli also stated that he found no evidence of publication bias in the ERUS literature in 2009.[14]

Niekel et al. reported no evidence of publication bias for M staging with CT,[15] but Dighe et al. reported that, for N staging with CT, evidence existed that smaller studies were reporting higher accuracies (suggesting publication bias), and a nonsignificant trend showed the same result for T staging.[16]

Niekel et al. reported that the MRI staging literature contained no evidence of publication bias.[15]

Too few studies are available for most of the evidence bases in this review to allow a statistical analysis of the possibility of publication bias. However, because of reports that the ERUS literature, in particular, may be affected by publication bias, we prepared funnel plots for the two larger ERUS evidence bases and also ran a metaregression against publication date. Although visual inspection of funnel plots is of limited value in determining the presence of publication bias, the plots look fairly symmetrical, and there does not appear to be any pattern by date in the ERUS-versus-CT evidence base. There may be a tendency to report higher accuracy in older studies in the MRI-versus-ERUS evidence base, but the number of studies in that evidence base is too small to allow us to reach any firm conclusion.

Key Question 2. What is the comparative effectiveness of imaging techniques for restaging cancer in patients with primary and recurrent colorectal cancer after initial treatment?

Key Question 2a. What is the test performance of the imaging techniques used (singly, in combination, or in a specific sequence) to restage colorectal cancer compared with a reference standard?

As noted previously, interim restaging takes place after neoadjuvant chemotherapy and/or radiotherapy and, in some cases, surgery. We identified only one recent (2009 or later) high-quality systematic review of interim restaging. Therefore, we searched for older high-quality systematic reviews of interim restaging but did not identify any that met the inclusion criteria. We identified nine primary comparative studies of interim restaging.

The one systematic review of interim restaging studied CT, MRI, and PET/CT for detecting liver metastases after neoadjuvant chemotherapy. The review authors concluded that MRI was more sensitive for this purpose than the other two modalities, but even for MRI the sensitivity was very low, possibly too low to be clinically useful (69.9%; 95% CI, 65.6% to 73.9%).

We identified four studies of interim rectal T staging. One study compared CT with MRI, one compared CT with ERUS, and two compared MRI, ERUS, and CT. Considering all the evidence in a qualitative fashion, the evidence seems to consistently support the conclusion that no significant difference in accuracy exists across ERUS, CT, and MRI for interim rectal T staging.

We identified three studies of interim rectal N restaging. One study compared ERUS with CT, and two studies compared ERUS, CT and MRI. There were no statistically significant differences across the modalities, but there was a nonsignificant trend for ERUS to be more accurate than MRI and CT and for MRI to be more accurate than CT.

We identified four studies of interim colorectal M restaging. Three compared MRI with CT, and one compared PET/CT with CT. We pooled the data reported by the three studies of MRI compared with CT for detecting liver metastases in a random-effects meta-analysis. The results indicated a nonsignificant trend toward MRI being more accurate in detecting colorectal liver metastases than CT.

No studies meeting inclusion criteria reported on interim colon cancer restaging separately (i.e., without mixing rectal cancer cases into the enrolled group), and no studies identified interim colorectal T and N restaging or interim rectal M restaging. We identified only one study of interim rectal CRM status.

Key Question 2b. What is the impact of alternative imaging techniques on intermediate outcomes, including stage reclassification and changes in therapeutic management?

No studies that met the inclusion criteria addressed this question.

Key Question 2c. What is the impact of alternative imaging techniques on clinical outcomes?

No studies that met the inclusion criteria addressed this question.

Key Question 2d. What are the adverse effects or harms associated with using imaging techniques, including harms of test-directed management?

See the answer to Key Question 1d for harms associated with any use of these imaging tests.

Key Question 2e. How is the comparative effectiveness of imaging techniques modified by the following factors:

  i. Patient-level characteristics (e.g., age, sex, body mass index)?
  ii. Disease characteristics (e.g., tumor grade)?
  iii. Imaging technique or protocol characteristics (e.g., use of different tracers or contrast agents, radiation dose of the imaging modality, slice thickness, timing of contrast)?

Only one study of MRI reported on factors affecting accuracy of interim N restaging, and only one study of MRI reported on factors affecting accuracy of interim M restaging.

Conclusions for Key Question 2

The one included systematic review reported that CT and PET/CT had sensitivities of approximately 50 percent for detecting colorectal liver metastases in the interim restaging setting, and MRI's sensitivity in this setting, although slightly better, is still quite low (69.9%; 95% CI, 65.6% to 73.9%).

We found no significant difference in accuracy across ERUS, CT, and MRI for interim rectal T staging and a nonsignificant trend for MRI to be more accurate than CT for detecting colorectal liver metastases during restaging.

The primary conclusion to be reached for Key Question 2 is that there are gaps in the research that has been published. The evidence base is small and limited. Only 10 studies addressed Key Question 2, all of which were rated as being at low to moderate risk of bias. The risk-of-bias rating by key factors is provided in Appendix D. There were too few studies to allow assessment of the possibility of publication bias.

Discussion

Key Findings and Strength of Evidence

Our major conclusions about comparative effectiveness are listed in Table E, along with the strength-of-evidence grade. We have moderate confidence in one conclusion and low confidence in several other conclusions, but the evidence was insufficient for the majority of the questions posed in this review.

Table E. Summary of major conclusions

Conclusion Statement	Strength of Evidence
ERUS is less likely to give an incorrect result (OR = 0.36; 95% CI, 0.24 to 0.54), less likely to understage (OR = 0.63; 95% CI, 0.44 to 0.89), and less likely to overstage (OR = 0.47; 95% CI, 0.28 to 0.80) rectal cancer than CT in the preoperative T staging setting.[a]	Low
MRI and ERUS are similar in accuracy for preoperative rectal T staging	Low
CT, MRI, and ERUS are similar in accuracy for preoperative rectal N staging. MRI is less likely than CT to overstage (OR = 0.498; 95% CI, 0.308 to 0.806).	Low
MRI is superior (more likely to detect lesions) to CT in detecting colorectal liver metastases in the preoperative setting (OR = 1.334; 95% CI, 1.012 to 1.761).[b]	Moderate
MRI, CT, and ERUS are similar in accuracy for rectal T staging in the interim restaging setting.	Low

[a] OR < 1 indicates a lower risk of error; OR > 1 indicates a higher risk of error.
[b] OR > 1 indicates a higher likelihood of detecting metastatic lesions.

CI = confidence interval; CT = computed tomography; ERUS = endorectal ultrasound; MRI = magnetic resonance imaging; N = nodal stage; OR = odds ratio; T = tumor stage.

For harms, in general, all four imaging modalities appear to be reasonably safe. For ERUS, the most common adverse event appears to be pain and minor bleeding; in theory, the major adverse event of bowel perforation could occur, but no included studies reported such an event. Our supplementary harms searches identified a narrative review of complications of endoscopic ultrasound, including ERUS.[17] The authors noted that only one case had been reported in a prospective registry of the German Society of Ultrasound in Medicine but did not report the number of ERUS procedures in the registry.

Harms from CT include contrast agent reactions and radiation exposure. Many of the included studies did not use intravenous contrast, and limited data suggest that using intravenous contrast does not improve the accuracy of CT for colorectal T or N staging. Not surprisingly, there were no studies comparing M staging by CT with and without contrast.

Harms from MRI appear to be limited to contrast agent reactions. Many of the included studies did not use intravenous contrast, and data suggest that the use of intravenous contrast does not improve MRI's accuracy for rectal T or N staging.

The major harm from PET/CT is radiation exposure. A single PET/CT examination exposes the patient to approximately 18 mSv, with the majority coming from the radiotracer for the PET component. Some experts believe this is a significant exposure; however, in 2010, the Health Physics Society published a position statement recommending against quantitative estimates of health risks below an individual dose of 5 rem per year (approximately 50 mSv) or a lifetime dose of 10 rem in addition to natural background radiation.[18] However, if a patient undergoes a PET/CT scan for staging, has surgical treatment, and then has regular CT scans for surveillance, the accumulated radiation dose could approach or exceed these limits.

Indirect harms of imaging primarily consist of harms related to incorrect treatment decisions based on inaccurate staging.

Limitations of the Evidence Base

The evidence base is quite limited. Very few studies reported on any outcomes other than staging accuracy. Among studies reporting only accuracy outcomes, we did not find complete cross-classifed data (i.e., numbers of patients correctly staged, understaged, and overstaged for each stage for all modalities and the reference standard). Many of the studies that reported on staging accuracy were quite small and provided limited information on patient characteristics. In particular, the evidence base for Key Question 2, interim restaging, is very sparse even for staging accuracy outcomes.

A few studies reported on how imaging modalities affected patient management, but few of these reported whether management changes were deemed appropriate. No studies reported on patient-oriented outcomes such as survival and quality of life.

Applicability

Judging the applicability of the results is difficult. The majority of studies reported very little information about patient characteristics. Most of the studies were set in university-based academic or teaching hospitals, which may limit the applicability of the results to community-based general hospitals. Another area of concern about applicability is the inclusion of many older studies that may have used technology that is now obsolete. During the topic refinement process, experts agreed that using an arbitrary publication cutoff date would introduce bias, so our literature searches went back to 1980.

Research Gaps

The majority of the evidence gaps on the questions in this review fall into the category of insufficient information.

There is practically no literature on interim restaging of either colon or rectal cancer, and very few studies of staging of colon cancer; most of the literature identified was about rectal cancer. This likely reflects the relatively greater importance of clinical locoregional staging in rectal versus colon cancer. Specifically, most studies of staging in colon cancer seemed to focus on looking for metastases, particularly to the liver.

Few studies examined the impact of combining different imaging modalities on pretreatment and interim staging assessments, which may provide more clinically relevant results than studies that examine the accuracy of one imaging modality in isolation. Given that patients often undergo multiple imaging studies for staging purposes, such information would be valuable.

Few studies addressed variations in imaging protocols that could affect study accuracy. Reviewers pointed out particular interest in factors that could affect accuracy of ERUS, such as the types of probes used and the experience of the individual performing the examination.

Very few studies of PET/CT are available; this is a concern because many experts appear to believe its addition to staging leads to useful changes in management. Also, its use for primary and interim clinical staging of patients is on the rise, despite the lack of convincing evidence to support its widespread adoption. We identified one study of changes in management after addition of PET/CT that concluded that only half of the changes in management triggered by PET/CT were appropriate, suggesting that using PET/CT for staging may result in significant patient harm.[19] Further study on this topic needs to be performed before any firm conclusions about the accuracy and clinical usefulness of PET/CT can be drawn.

Not having the right information is another consideration. Insufficient information is available about changes in management triggered by imaging studies and about patient-oriented outcomes downstream of staging. Ideally, randomized controlled trials would be designed to test different staging and management strategies, capturing health outcomes that occur following treatment.

Studies of the impact of imaging on patient management decisions are potentially helpful and can be accomplished in shorter timeframes than studies measuring health outcomes. However, it is critical to confirm whether the changes in management were appropriate; simply reporting that adding information from an imaging modality led to changes in management is insufficient information to be clinically useful.

Conclusions

Low-strength evidence suggests ERUS is more accurate than CT for preoperative rectal cancer T staging and MRI is similar in accuracy to ERUS. Moderate-strength evidence suggests MRI is superior to CT for detecting colorectal liver metastases. There was insufficient evidence to come to any evidence-based conclusions about the use of PET/CT for colorectal cancer staging. Low-strength evidence suggests that CT, MRI, and ERUS are comparable for rectal cancer N staging, but all are limited in sensitivity. Low-strength evidence suggests that they are also comparable for interim rectal cancer T restaging, but both sensitivity and specificity are suboptimal. While all four imaging modalities appear to be reasonably safe, long-range harm from radiation exposure over repeated examinations is particularly of concern with PET/CT.

References

1. American Cancer Society. Cancer Facts & Figures 2012. Atlanta; 2012. www.cancer.org/acs/groups/content/@epidemiologysurveilance/documents/document/acspc-031941.pdf.

2. American Cancer Society. Colorectal cancer Facts & Figures 2011-2013. Atlanta; 2011. www.cancer.org/acs/groups/content/@epidemiologysurveilance/documents/document/acspc-028323.pdf.

3. Yabroff KR, Lund J, Kepka D, et al. Economic burden of cancer in the United States: estimates, projections, and future research. Cancer Epidemiol Biomarkers Prev. 2011 Oct;20(10):2006-14. PMID: 21980008.

4. Mariotto AB, Yabroff KR, Shao Y, et al. Projections of the cost of cancer care in the United States: 2010-2020. J Natl Cancer Inst. 2011 Jan 19;103(2):117-28. PMID: 21228314.

5. U.S. Preventive Services Task Force. Screening for Colorectal Cancer. March 2009. www.uspreventiveservicestaskforce.org/uspstf/uspscolo.htm. Accessed January 23, 2014.

6. White CM, Ip S, McPheeters M, et al. Using existing systematic reviews to replace de novo processes in conducting Comparative Effectiveness Reviews. Sept. 2009. In: Methods Guide for Effectiveness and Comparative Effectiveness Reviews. AHRQ Publication No. 10(14)-EHC063-EF. Rockville, MD: Agency for Healthcare Research and Quality. January 2014. Chapters available at www.effectivehealthcare.ahrq.gov. PMID: 21433402.

7. Owens DK, Lohr KN, Atkins D, et al. Grading the strength of a body of evidence when comparing medical interventions-Agency for Healthcare Research and Quality and the Effective Health Care Program. J Clin Epidemiol. 2010 May;63(5):513-23. PMID: 19595577.

8. Owens D, Lohr K, Atkins D, et al. Grading the strength of a body of evidence when comparing medical interventions. July 2009. In: Methods Guide for Effectiveness and Comparative Effectiveness Reviews. AHRQ Publication No. 10(14)-EHC063-EF. Rockville, MD: Agency for Healthcare Research and Quality. January 2014. Chapters available at www.effectivehealthcare.ahrq.gov.

9. Methods Guide for Medical Test Reviews. AHRQ Publication No. 12-EHC017. Rockville, MD: Agency for Healthcare Research and Quality; June 2012. www://effectivehealthcare.ahrq.gov/reports/final.cfm.

10. Harbord RM, Deeks JJ, Egger M, et al. A unification of models for meta-analysis of diagnostic accuracy studies. Biostatistics. 2007 Apr;8(2):239-51. PMID: 16698768.

11. STATA Statistics/Data Analysis. MP Parallel Edition. College Station, TX: StataCorp; 1984-2007. Single user Stata for Windows. www.stata.com.

12. Zamora J, Abraira V, Muriel A, et al. Meta-DiSc: a software for meta-analysis of test accuracy data. BMC Med Res Methodol. 2006;6:31. PMID: 16836745.

13. Harewood GC. Assessment of publication bias in the reporting of EUS performance in staging rectal cancer. Am J Gastroenterol. 2005 Apr;100(4):808-16. PMID: 15784023.

14. Puli SR, Bechtold ML, Reddy JB, et al. How good is endoscopic ultrasound in differentiating various T stages of rectal cancer? Meta-analysis and systematic review. Ann Surg Oncol. 2009 Feb;16(2):254-65. PMID: 19018597.

15. Niekel MC, Bipat S, Stoker J. Diagnostic imaging of colorectal liver metastases with CT, MR imaging, FDG PET, and/or FDG PET/CT: a meta-analysis of prospective studies including patients who have not previously undergone treatment. Radiology. 2010 Dec;257(3):674-84. PMID: 20829538.

16. Dighe S, Purkayastha S, Swift I, et al. Diagnostic precision of CT in local staging of colon cancers: a meta-analysis. Clin Radiol. 2010 Sep;65(9):708-19. PMID: 20696298.

17. Jenssen C, Alvarez-Sanchez MV, Napoleon B, et al. Diagnostic endoscopic ultrasonography: assessment of safety and prevention of complication. World J Gastroenterol. 2012 Sep 14;18(34):4659-76. PMID: 23002335.

18. Radiation Risk in Perspective. Position Statement of the Health Physics Society. McLean, VA: Health Physics Society; July 2010. http://hps.org/documents/risk_ps010-2.pdf

19. Ramos E, Valls C, Martinez L, et al. Preoperative staging of patients with liver metastases of colorectal carcinoma. Does PET/CT really add something to multidetector CT? Ann Surg Oncol. 2011 Sep;18(9):2654-61. PMID: 21431987.

Introduction

Background

Colorectal Cancer

In the United States, colon cancer is diagnosed in approximately 100,000 patients and rectal cancer is diagnosed in another 50,000 each year.[1] These cancers most commonly affect older adults, with 90 percent of cases diagnosed in individuals older than 50 years.[2] Colorectal cancer is often fatal, with approximately 50,000 deaths attributed to it each year in the United States.[1] As such, it is the third-most common type of cancer and the third-most common cause of cancer-related death for both men and women. Colorectal cancer is also associated with high health care costs. It has been estimated to be the cancer site with the second-highest associated cost of care (second only to female breast cancer).[3,4]

Ninety-six percent of colorectal cancers are epithelial adenocarcinomas,[20] which develop from the cells that line the interior of the colon and rectum (the large intestine). The large intestine is the final segment of the digestive tract, and its primary function in digestion is to extract water and minerals from the remaining food matter and then store the resulting solid waste in the rectum until it can be excreted. The colon consists of four sections: the ascending colon, which is attached to the small intestine and loops upward on the right side of the abdomen; the transverse colon, which passes horizontally from the right to the left side of the abdomen; the descending colon, which passes downward on the left side of the abdomen; and the sigmoid colon, which is S-shaped and attaches to the rectum.

Most colorectal cancers develop slowly over decades.[21] The process involves a gradual accumulation of genetic mutations and epigenetic alterations. The first histologically detectable change is development of aberrant crypt foci in the lining of the intestine. The crypt foci may progress to adenomatous polyps, some of which (an estimated 10 percent) may eventually progress to invasive cancer (adenocarcinomas). Adenomatous polyps are very common, possibly affecting 50 percent of the population. Many individuals form more than one polyp.[22] Removing screening-detected polyps may prevent colorectal cancer from forming.[23]

Although often mentioned together as if they were the same condition, colon and rectal cancer differ significantly in their epidemiology, prognosis, and treatment. Colon cancer is more common than rectal cancer and can be subdivided as proximal (involving the cecum, ascending, and transverse colon) or distal (involving the descending and sigmoid colon) cancer. Men are more likely to develop distal colon and rectal cancer, and women and younger patients of either sex are more likely to develop proximal colon cancer.[24,25]

Risk factors for developing colorectal cancer include a family history of colorectal cancer or adenomatous polyps, a personal history of chronic inflammatory bowel disease, physical inactivity, obesity, frequent consumption of red meat that has been cooked at a high temperature or for a long time, frequent consumption of processed preserved meats, smoking, and heavy alcohol consumption.[2] Regular use of nonsteroidal anti-inflammatory drugs (NSAIDs) may reduce the risk of colorectal cancer, as does the use of postmenopausal hormonal replacement therapy.[2] About 5 percent of individuals in whom colorectal cancer has been diagnosed have a well-defined genetic syndrome, such as hereditary nonpolyposis colorectal cancer (Lynch syndrome) or familial adenomatous polyposis.[2]

Colorectal cancers may be diagnosed during screening of asymptomatic individuals or after the patient has developed symptoms. Colon cancer symptoms can include abdominal discomfort, change in bowel habits (diarrhea or constipation), fatigue due to anemia, and weight loss. Rectal cancer symptoms include bleeding, diarrhea, and pain. The United States Preventive Services Task Force currently recommends screening for colorectal cancer in asymptomatic individuals using fecal occult blood testing, sigmoidoscopy, or colonoscopy, beginning at age 50 years and continuing until age 75 years.[5] Diagnosis is usually established through histopathologic examination of tissue samples (obtained through colonoscopy or biopsy).

Staging

Staging Systems

Once the diagnosis has been established, patients with colorectal cancer undergo testing to establish the extent of disease spread, known as clinical staging. Staging is used primarily to determine appropriate treatment strategies. Staging consists of assessing the status of the tumor in regards to various factors, such as depth of tumor invasion into the colorectal wall, fat and fascia involvement, status of circumferential resection margin, invasion into surrounding structures, involvement of local lymph nodes, and distant metastasis. Determining the correct clinical stage for colon and rectal cancer is of the utmost importance because treatment options differ greatly depending on the clinical stage of disease at diagnosis; for example, tumors confined to the rectal wall can be treated by local excision, but tumors that have progressed to involve the fascia and fat usually require preoperative chemotherapy and radiation prior to surgical resection. Similarly, the presence of distant metastases usually leads to a decision to use chemotherapy rather than surgical resection. Stage is not the only determinant of treatment options; patient comorbidities and preferences and clinician and institution preferences are also used in decisionmaking. However, stage is the key determinant of the management strategy. Staging is also used to inform patient prognosis and identify patients at higher risk of relapse or cancer-related mortality.

The American Joint Committee on Cancer (AJCC) endorses the widely accepted "TNM" staging system for colorectal cancer. This system is consistent with the Union for International Cancer Control staging system, allowing direct comparisons across clinical research centers or countries. The AJCC system aims to characterize the anatomic extent of colorectal cancer based on three tumor characteristics: the extent of tumor infiltration into the bowel wall (tumor stage, designated as "T"), the extent of local or regional lymph node spread (nodal stage, designated as "N"), and the presence of distant metastatic lesions (metastatic spread, designated as "M").

Once the T, N, and M components are determined, they are used to assign the disease into four broad stages of increasingly unfavorable prognosis (denoted I through IV). The categories are mutually exclusive (i.e., a patient can belong to only one category) and exhaustive (i.e., all patients belong to a category). Two other, older colorectal cancer staging systems—the Dukes[26] and modified Astler-Coller[27] staging systems—are less widely used. One of the challenges we had to overcome in this systematic review was determining how cancer stages can be translated between staging systems or within versions of the AJCC staging system, currently in its 7th edition. The 5th edition was released in 1998, the 6th edition in 2003, and the 7th edition in 2010. The major difference between the 5th/6th systems and the 7th system is the earlier versions do not separate stage T4 into subgroups, do not separate stage N1/N2 into subgroups, and do not separate stage M1 into subgroups. The staging systems are summarized below, in Table 1 through Table 4.

Besides the factors considered in the TNM system, the circumferential resection margin is an important indicator of prognosis and essential information for treatment planning for rectal cancer.[28,29] The circumferential resection margin is defined as the distance from the edge of the tumor to the margin of the resected specimen. Imaging technologies such as magnetic resonance imaging (MRI) are capable of predicting tumor involvement of the surgical circumferential resection margin. Patients with positive margins are at much higher risk of recurrence (19 percent to 22 percent vs. 3 percent to 5 percent risk for those with negative margins).[28]

The depth of tumor invasion outside the muscularis propria is also thought to be an important factor to consider in rectal cancer staging. The 5-year survival rate drops from 85 percent to 54 percent when the depth of tumor invasion outside the muscularis propria exceeds 5 mm.[30] The Radiological Society of North American suggests modifying the T3 stage by adding a letter that describes the depth of invasion (namely, T3a is less than 5 mm of invasion; T3b is 5–10 mm of invasion; T3c is more than 10 mm of invasion).[30]

Table 1. Tumor-Node-Metastasis (TNM) definitions for colorectal cancer

T	N	M
Tx: No description of the tumor's extent is possible because of incomplete information. **Tis:** The cancer is in the earliest stage (in situ). It involves only the mucosa. It has not grown beyond the muscularis mucosa (inner muscle layer). **T1:** The cancer has grown through the muscularis mucosa and extends into the submucosa. **T2:** The cancer has grown through the submucosa and extends into the muscularis propria (thick outer muscle layer). **T3:** The cancer has grown through the muscularis propria and into the outermost layers of the colon or rectum but not through them. It has not reached any nearby organs or tissues. **T4a:** The cancer has grown through the serosa (also known as the visceral peritoneum), the outermost lining of the intestines. **T4b:** The cancer has grown through the wall of the colon or rectum and is attached to or invades into nearby tissues or organs.	**Nx:** No description of lymph node involvement is possible because of incomplete information. **N0:** No cancer in nearby lymph nodes. **N1:** Cancer cells are found in or near 1 to 3 nearby lymph nodes **N1a:** Cancer cells are found in 1 nearby lymph node. **N1b:** Cancer cells are found in 2–3 nearby lymph nodes. **N1c:** Small deposits of cancer cells are found in areas of fat near lymph nodes, but not in the lymph nodes themselves. **N2:** Cancer cells are found in 4 or more nearby lymph nodes **N2a:** Cancer cells are found in 4–6 nearby lymph nodes. **N2b:** Cancer cells are found in 7 or more nearby lymph nodes.	**M0:** No distant spread is seen. **M1a:** The cancer has spread to 1 distant organ or set of distant lymph nodes. **M1b:** The cancer has spread to more than 1 distant organ or set of distant lymph nodes, or it has spread to distant parts of the peritoneum (the lining of the abdominal cavity).

T: Categories of colorectal cancer describe the extent of spread through the layers that form the wall of the colon and rectum.
N: Categories indicate whether or not the cancer has spread to nearby lymph nodes and, if so, how many lymph nodes are involved.
M: Categories indicate whether or not the cancer has spread (metastasized) to distant organs, such as the liver, lungs, or distant lymph nodes.

Table 2. Dukes system

A	Tumor confined to the intestinal wall
B	Tumor invading through the intestinal wall
C1	With lymph node involvement, but not apical node
C2	With lymph node involvement, including apical node
D	Distant metastasis

Table 3. Modified Astler-Coller system

A	Tumor limited to mucosa
B1	Tumor invading into muscularis
B2	Tumor invading into serosa
B3	Tumor invading into adjacent organs
C1, C2, C3	Relevant B category but with lymph node involvement
D	Distant metastasis

Table 4. Taxonomic and prognostic groups based on the AJCC, Dukes, and Modified Astler-Coller staging systems

Stage	T	N	M	Dukes	MAC
0	Tis	N0	M0	—	—
I	T1	N0	M0	A	A
	T2	N0	M0	A	B1
IIA	T3	N0	M0	B	B2
IIB	T4a	N0	M0	B	B2
IIC	T4b	N0	M0	B	B3
IIIA	T1-T2	N1/N1c	M0	C	C1
	T1	N2a	M0	C	C1
IIIB	T3-T4a	N1/N1c	M0	C	C2
	T2-T3	N2a	M0	C	C1/C2
	T1-T2	N2b	M0	C	C1
IIIC	T4a	N2a	M0	C	C2
	T3-T4a	N2b	M0	C	C2
	T4b	N1-N2	M0	C	C3
IVA	Any T	Any N	M1a	D	D
IVB	Any T	Any N	M1b	D	D

MAC=Modified Astler-Coller system; T=tumor stage; N=nodal stage'. M=distant metastasis stage

Staging/Interim Restaging

Staging is performed at two distinct time points in managing colorectal cancer. The first is immediately after diagnosis, before any treatment has been given. Imaging and clinical examination are used to assign the clinical stage, which is used to make decisions about primary treatment and management. The second time point applies only to patients who, on the basis of their primary clinical stage, were treated with neoadjuvant chemotherapy or radiotherapy instead of with immediate surgery. For clinical stage I colon or rectal cancer and clinical stage II, or III colon cancer, surgical resection is the primary treatment. For patients with clinical stage II or III rectal cancer, preoperative chemotherapy and possibly radiation is the preferred initial treatment. Surgery is an option for some patients with clinical stage IV colorectal cancer, but for these patients, primary treatment is chemotherapy.[31]

Clinical staging after initial treatment with chemotherapy and radiotherapy (interim staging or restaging) is primarily intended to determine whether the tumor has responded to the initial treatment (downstaging). Chemotherapy and radiotherapy affect the metabolism and structure of the tissues such that some kinds of imaging may be less accurate for restaging than in the pretreatment setting. Also, the role of imaging at each of these two time points is very different, and for these two reasons they are addressed in separate key questions in this review.

Recurrent Colorectal Cancer

Recurrent colorectal cancer arises in some patients after undergoing apparently successful initial treatment for primary colorectal cancer. Approximately 20 to 30 percent of patients will develop recurrent disease. After completing primary treatment, patients usually enter a routine surveillance program intended to detect signs of recurrence. Typically, this consists of regular tests for biomarkers (such as carcinoembryonic antigen), clinical examination, colonoscopies, and possibly computed tomography (CT) scans.[31] After the diagnosis of a possible recurrence, clinical staging aims to assess the extent of disease to guide treatment decisions and determine prognosis. Multiple treatment options (e.g., chemotherapy alone vs. multimodality therapy, including metastasectomy) are available for patients with recurrent disease, and the decision is chiefly based on accurate clinical assessment of the extent of disease.[31]

Imaging Technologies

Imaging tests can be broadly divided into two categories: some tests primarily provide anatomic information (e.g., CT), whereas others primarily provide functional information in terms of metabolic activity (e.g., positron emission tomography [PET]). An important characteristic of imaging tests to consider is whether they use ionizing radiation; for patients with colorectal cancer who have a long life expectancy (e.g., those with early-stage disease who undergo treatment with curative intent), the cumulative exposure to ionizing radiation during diagnosis, staging, and subsequent surveillance can be substantial.[32]

Different imaging tests provide different information for assessing TNM stage. For example, endoscopic ultrasound can provide information on the "local stage" (i.e., the depth of invasion of the cancer into the bowel wall), but not on the presence of distant metastases. In contrast, whole-body CT or PET/CT may not be useful for assessing depth of invasion into the bowel wall, but can provide information on metastatic lesions, even when patients have no symptoms from the lesions. Consequently, no single test may be sufficient for staging, and different combinations of tests are possible.

In the following sections, we discuss endoscopic ultrasound, CT, MRI, and PET/CT techniques.

Endoscopic Ultrasound

Endoscopic ultrasound (also referred to as endorectal ultrasound, or endoscopic rectal ultrasound) entered into clinical practice for staging rectal cancer in the early 1980s. As the ultrasound probe is inserted into the rectum and can only visualize the immediate area around the rectum, it is only able to assess the clinical T and N stages (not distant metastatic disease).

The procedure requires an empty rectum, which can be achieved by using standard bowel preparation protocols developed for colonoscopy or laxative enemas. The patient usually does not need to be sedated. Three different types of equipment are commonly used: flexible echoendoscopes, rigid probes with a radial transducer, and high-frequency miniprobes inside standard endoscopes. Variable ultrasound frequencies (5–15 MHz) are used because higher frequencies provide better resolution of the rectal wall, but lower frequencies are better for visualizing lymph nodes and perirectal tissue.[33] ERUS is not suitable for use in patients with stenosing tumors, as it may be impossible to advance the probe beyond the tumor.

One of the problems with ERUS is that image quality and interpretation is primarily done by visually inspecting the image. Thus, the diagnostic accuracy varies with the operator's skill and experience level.[33] Burtin et al. reported that interobserver agreement was particularly poor for staging T2 rectal tumors.[34]

Ultrasound employs high-frequency sound waves that reflect at boundaries between tissues with different acoustic properties. B-mode gray-scale ultrasound is the most commonly used type of ultrasound.[35] This mode uses differences in the reflection and absorption of sound waves by different tissue types to visualize internal anatomy. The contrast resolution of conventional ultrasound depends distance from the transducer to the structures of interest as well as on the transducer's frequency. Advanced software programs using three-dimensional (3D) reconstruction of the anatomy are becoming more commonly used and may improve recognition of the rectal anatomy and pathologic lesions.[36]

Doppler ultrasound evaluates blood flow through vessels by observing changes in the pitch of the reflected sound waves (the Doppler effect). Doppler can be helpful when evaluating soft tissue masses because malignant masses usually demonstrate increased vascularity compared with benign tissues. Doppler imaging can also be performed with microbubble contrast agents that enhance evaluation of the vascularity of soft tissue masses which can be helpful in distinguishing between malignancy and benign lesions.[37]

Two primary types of Doppler imaging exist: color and power. Color Doppler imaging encodes the mean Doppler frequency shifts at particular locations in various colors, whereas power Doppler imaging encodes the power of the signal (extent of the Doppler effect) at particular locations in various colors.[38] Color Doppler, therefore, detects the velocity of the blood cells, and power Doppler detects the amount of blood present.[38]

The American College of Radiology (ACR) has instituted a voluntary general ultrasound accreditation program that offers facilities the opportunity for peer review of their staff qualifications, equipment, and quality control and quality-assurance programs.[39]

Magnetic Resonance Imaging

MRI systems use strong magnetic fields and radiofrequency energy to translate hydrogen nuclei distribution in tissues into computer-generated images of the body. MRI does not expose patients to radiation, but does often involve the use of contrast agents to improve image resolution.

MRI systems are usually described primarily in terms of magnet strength, in the unit tesla (T). Systems in commercial use usually vary from 0.5 T to 3.0 T. In general, increasing the magnet strength increases the spatial resolution of the images. MRI systems that use field strengths below 1 T are usually open gantries and are primarily used for patients who cannot be accommodated inside the bore of a higher-field-strength magnet because of claustrophobia. An additional reason to use open gantry systems is that MRI-guided invasive procedures, such as biopsies, are much easier to perform in open gantries than in closed systems.[40]

Special coils are routinely used in MRI to increase the efficiency of signal detection and, by extension, the image quality. At one time, endorectal coils were in common use, but problems with these coils (e.g., limited field of view, patient discomfort, difficulty in placing coils in patients with high or stenosing tumors) led to their abandonment in favor of dedicated surface phased array coils. Phased-array coils contain multiple surface coils that increase the signal-to-noise ratio and provide a large field of view with a high spatial resolution.[41]

Many different imaging protocols can be used on any MRI device, but most anatomic imaging protocols utilize. T1- or T2-weighted pulse sequences. Diffusion-weighted imaging, which measures the movement of water in the tissue, is a commonly performed functional imaging protocol.[42,43] While all suppliers of MRI equipment provide suggested protocols for different examination types, users commonly customize these. The degree of protocol customization largely depends on the clinical users, both radiologists and technologists. Even in well-run multi-institutional studies with a limited number of institutions all using equipment supplied by the same manufacturer, differences in technique have been observed.[44]

MR images are susceptible to a number of artifacts that could cause image distortion and false interpretations. Respiratory motion can be a problem, although when the patient is prone the effect is reduced.[45] MRI interpretation requires specialized training.[46,47] The accuracy of MR imaging depends on the image reader's experience and skill and is subject to significant inter- and intraobserver variability.[30] Computer-assisted imaging devices may reduce subjectivity and decrease time required for image interpretation.[48]

Gadolinium-based paramagnetic contrast agents accumulate in the vascular system and can aid in tumor visualization by highlighting areas of increased vascularity through differential enhancement. Five slightly different gadolinium-based contrast agents are in common clinical use: gadobenate dimeglumine, gadopentetate dimeglumine, gadodiamide, gadoteridol, and gadoversetamide.[49] Besides these general-purpose contrast agents, hepatobiliary-specific contrast agents are available for imaging the liver (e.g., gadoxetic acid).[50] These agents differ slightly in molecular structure; however, all consist of the heavy metal gadolinium bound to a chelating molecule.[51] Different agents demonstrate different imaging properties.[52,53] The exact dose of conventional gadolinium contrast agents is not particularly relevant to image quality when used in the normal range (0.1 to 0.2 mmol/kg). When contrast is taken up by a lesion, one of three characteristic enhancement and wash-out curves are usually observed: continuous enhancement, rapid enhancement followed by a plateau, or rapid enhancement followed by rapid wash-out. Rapid wash-out is considered indicative of malignancy.[46] However, many centers do not use intravenous contrast agents for rectal cancer staging because of the perception that it is not helpful.[54]

For rectal imaging, a contrast agent such as air, water, barium, ferumoxsil, or ultrasound gel may be introduced into the rectum through the anal sphincter after cleansing the rectum by enema.[30,54] The patient may be treated with an antispasmodic agent before imaging to reduce bowel motion.[54]

No nationwide compulsory accreditation exists for MRI facilities. ACR administers a voluntary accreditation program.[55]

Computed Tomography

CT uses x-rays to generate images of internal anatomy. In CT scanning, an x-ray source rotates around the body, scanning narrow "slices" of the body. As the x-rays pass through the body, they are absorbed differentially by different tissues. Opposite the x-ray source are detectors that collect the x-rays that have passed through the "slice" of body. The information collected by the detectors is used to generate images of the internal anatomy. Modern CT machines can scan in both axial and spiral fashion and have multiple detectors to collect information from multiple "slices" of the body simultaneously. As a result, CT examinations are typically performed in a single breath-hold, which reduces artifacts caused by respiratory and organ motion. In addition, with the use of thin section imaging, coronal and sagittal reformats can be generated from the axial images with good resolution; therefore aiding in the localization of primary tumor as well as identification of lymph nodes and metastatic lesions.

Iodinated contrast agents are sometimes used to enhance CT imaging of the vasculature. Intravenous contrast is typically used for staging colorectal cancer as it improves visualization of the tumor, lymph nodes, and metastatic lesions. Oral contrast agents are almost always used as well for staging examinations, as they help to differentiate the bowel from adjacent structures. Another option is to inflate the rectum with air or water to improve contrast.

ACR offers a voluntary accreditation program for CT facilities.[56]

Positron Emission Tomography/Computed Tomography

PET is a nuclear imaging modality that uses radioactive tracers to provide images reflecting metabolic processes. Several different radiopharmaceuticals can be used in PET imaging. The tracer most commonly used is ^{18}F-fluorodeoxyglucose (FDG), a glucose analog that accumulates in tissue in proportion to the metabolic activity of the tissue. The uptake of the radioactive tracer can be monitored by PET and provide images of regional glucose metabolism. Since rapidly dividing tumor cells metabolize large amounts of glucose. Areas of elevated metabolism, which may be tumor cells, can be visualized on the PET images. However, infected and inflamed tissue also take up FDG and can cause false-positive results; this can be a particular problem after radiation therapy, when tissues may exhibit a protracted inflammatory response.[57]

Stand-alone, whole-body PET scanners for oncology indications are rapidly becoming obsolete.[58] Combined CT/PET systems are increasingly available and account for almost all the new whole-body PET installations. In this report, we discuss whole-body scanners that combine PET with CT and not stand-alone PET scanners. These systems allow images of metabolism and anatomy to be obtained at the same time. When performing a PET/CT scan, a small amount of FDG is injected into the patient's bloodstream, and the device first performs a CT scan, which provides anatomic information, followed immediately by a PET scan, which provides metabolic information, highlighting areas of high tracer uptake. Whole-body scanners have a ring of detectors that surround the patient and can image the entire body. The 3D anatomic images (CT scanning) are overlaid over the PET images of metabolism on a computer workstation.

The standardized uptake value, which is the mean tracer activity detected normalized for the injected dose of tracer and patient's body weight, depends on an image reconstruction algorithm, which varies by device manufacturer.[59] Therefore, diagnostic performance of PET/CT imaging may vary across manufacturers. Diagnostic performance may also vary depending on study-specific factors such as FDG uptake time, patient motion, the size and histology of the lesion(s), patient weight, position and blood glucose level, spatial resolution, and interpretation of the final image.[60-62] PET images have a spatial resolution of 4 to 10 mm, limiting detection of very small lesions.[57]

The Intersocietal Accreditation Commission (formerly the Intersocietal Commission for the Accreditation of Nuclear Medicine Laboratories) offers voluntary accreditation to PET/CT facilities based on a peer review of their staff qualifications, education, equipment, quality control, and volume of clinical procedures.[63]

Scope and Key Questions

Scope of the Review

We have summarized key recommendations from organizations in the United States regarding the use of imaging tests for staging in Table 5. As the table shows, the organizations are not in complete agreement about which modalities should be emphasized for the clinical situations described. Also, no consensus guidance exists about the sequence in which these tests are to be applied in the staging process.

The imaging modalities vary in accuracy as well as in the harms they can potentially cause. To be clinically useful and relevant, these benefits should be weighed against the potential harms of using the modality. The tumor's size may also have a significant effect on the accuracy of the imaging modality. For example, the ACR guidelines[64] provide different recommendations for large and small rectal cancer lesions, whereas the National Comprehensive Cancer Network guidelines[31] do not make that distinction. The differences in the testing protocols associated with different imaging modalities can affect their test performance and need to be systematically reviewed. Although it is necessary to identify the most accurate test (or combination of tests) for correctly staging the cancer, it is also important to assess the relative impact of testing strategies using different imaging modalities on intermediate outcomes such as stage reclassification (i.e., an indication of how much additional information is obtained by applying a test) and therapeutic decisionmaking (i.e., measures of the impact of tests on clinical decisions), and clinical outcomes. Building on the available scientific data, it is hoped that this systematic review of the available imaging modalities for colorectal cancer staging will uncover evidence to support these questions or highlight any issues not addressed by the currently available evidence that may represent targets for future research.

More accurate staging of colorectal cancer allows clinicians to select more appropriate treatment options. Selection of more appropriate treatment options would be expected to improve clinical outcomes (e.g., by avoiding unnecessarily aggressive treatments for low-risk disease). Besides assisting in treatment selection, staging also provides important prognostic information about chances of short- and long-term survival.

This review's primary objective is to synthesize the available information on using imaging for staging colorectal cancer. The availability of this information will assist clinicians in selecting protocols for staging, may reduce variability across treatment centers in staging protocols, and may improve patient outcomes. A secondary objective is to identify gaps in the evidence base to inform future research needs.

Table 5. Summary of existing guidelines for staging colorectal cancer

Clinical Description	ACR Recommendations	NCCN Recommendations
Colon cancer	*Usually appropriate* • CT chest-abdomen-pelvis with or without contrast • X-ray chest (if chest CT is not performed) • FDG-PET whole body • MRI abdomen and pelvis with or without contrast	*Recommended* • Chest/abdominal/pelvic CT with IV and oral contrast
	May be appropriate • MRI abdomen and pelvis without contrast • CT chest-abdomen-pelvis with and without contrast • CT chest-abdomen-pelvis without contrast	
	Usually not appropriate None reported	*Usually not indicated* PET scan PET-CT does not supplant a contrast-enhanced diagnostic CT

Table 5. Summary of existing guidelines for staging colorectal cancer (continued)

Clinical Description	ACR Recommendations	NCCN Recommendations

Rectal cancer	*Usually appropriate for small lesions*
	  US pelvis endorectal
	  X-ray chest (if chest is not imaged by CT)
	  CT chest-abdomen-pelvis with or without contrast
	  MRI pelvis with or without contrast
	
	Usually appropriate for large lesions
	  X-ray chest
	  CT chest-abdomen-pelvis with or without contrast
	  MRI abdomen with or without contrast
	  MRI pelvis with or without contrast
	  FDG-PET whole body
		Recommended
		  Chest/abdominal/pelvic CT
		  Endorectal US or endorectal/pelvic MRI

	May be appropriate for small lesions
	  FDG-PET whole body
	  MRI abdomen with and without contrast
	  MRI abdomen without contrast
	  CT chest-abdomen-pelvis without contrast
	  CT chest-abdomen-pelvis with and without contrast
	  MRI pelvis without contrast
	
	May be appropriate for large lesions
	  US pelvis endorectal
	  MRI abdomen without contrast
	  MRI abdomen with contrast
	  CT chest-abdomen-pelvis without contrast
	  CT chest-abdomen-pelvis with and without contrast	

	Usually not appropriate
	  None reported
		Usually not indicated
		  PET-CT not routinely indicated

Suspected liver metastases following detection of primary tumor[65]	*Usually appropriate*
	  CT abdomen with contrast
	  MRI abdomen with and without contrast
	  FDG-PET skull base to mid-thigh
	
	May be appropriate
	  MRI abdomen without contrast
	  CT abdomen with and without contrast
	  CT abdomen without contrast
	  US abdomen
	
	Usually not appropriate
	  CTA abdomen with contrast
	  In-111 somatostatin receptor scintigraphy	

Table 5. Summary of existing guidelines for staging colorectal cancer (continued)

Clinical Description	ACR Recommendations	NCCN Recommendations
Suspected or proven metastatic synchronous adenocarcinoma (M1)		*Recommended* Chest/abdominal/pelvic CT (with IV contrast); Consider MRI with IV contrast if CT is inadequate Needle biopsy (if indicated) *May be appropriate* PET-CT scan only if potentially curable M1 disease

ACR=American College of Radiology; CT=computed tomography; CTA=computed tomography angiography; FDG=[18]F-fluorodeoxyglucose tracer with positron emission tomography; IV=intravenous; MRI=magnetic resonance imaging; NCCN=National Comprehensive Cancer Network; PET=positron emission tomography; PET-CT=positron emission tomography combined with computerized tomography; US=ultrasonography.

Key Questions

The draft key questions were posted for public comment in November 2012 on the Web site of the Effective Health Care Program. No comments were received; therefore, no substantive changes were made to the key questions. They are listed below:

Key Question 1. What is the comparative effectiveness of imaging techniques for pretreatment cancer staging in patients with primary and recurrent colorectal cancer?

   a. What is the test performance of the imaging techniques used (singly, in combination, or in a specific sequence) to stage colorectal cancer compared with a reference standard?
   b. What is the impact of alternative imaging techniques on intermediate outcomes, including stage reclassification and changes in therapeutic management?
   c. What is the impact of alternative imaging techniques on clinical outcomes?
   d. What are the adverse effects or harms associated with using imaging techniques, including harms of test-directed management?
   e. How is the comparative effectiveness of imaging techniques modified by the following factors:
       i. Patient-level characteristics (e.g., age, sex, body mass index)
       ii. Disease characteristics (e.g., tumor grade)
       iii. Imaging technique or protocol characteristics (e.g., use of different tracers or contrast agents, radiation dose of the imaging modality, slice thickness, timing of contrast)

Key Question 2. What is the comparative effectiveness of imaging techniques for restaging cancer in patients with primary and recurrent colorectal cancer after initial treatment?

   a. What is the test performance of the imaging techniques used (singly, in combination, or in a specific sequence) to restage colorectal cancer compared with a reference standard?
   b. What is the impact of alternative imaging techniques on intermediate outcomes, including stage reclassification and changes in therapeutic management?
   c. What is the impact of alternative imaging techniques on clinical outcomes?
   d. What are the adverse effects or harms associated with using imaging techniques, including harms of test-directed management?
   e. How is the comparative effectiveness of imaging techniques modified by the following factors:
       i. Patient-level characteristics (e.g., age, sex, body mass index)
       ii. Disease characteristics (e.g., tumor grade)
       iii. Imaging technique or protocol characteristics (e.g., use of different tracers or contrast agents, radiation dose of the imaging modality, slice thickness, timing of contrast)

PICOTS

Populations:
- Adult patients with an established diagnosis of primary colorectal cancer
- Adult patients with an established diagnosis of recurrent colorectal cancer

Interventions:

Noninvasive imaging using the following tests (alone or in combination) for assessing the stage of colorectal cancer:
- Computed tomography (CT)
- Positron emission tomography combined with computerized tomography (PET/CT)
- Magnetic resonance imaging (MRI)
- Endoscopic rectal ultrasound (ERUS

Reference Standards to Assess Test Performance:
- Histopathologic examination of tissue
- Intraoperative findings
- Clinical followup

Histopathology of surgically resected specimens is the reference standard for pretherapy staging. In patients undergoing surgery, the nodal stage and spread of the tumor to nearby regional structures and other organs are assessed intraoperatively either by palpation or ultrasound. However, in patients with metastatic disease who undergo palliative care, a combination of initial biopsy results and clinical followup serves as the reference standard. The results from the imaging modality or modalities are used to arrive at a stage determination that is compared against the stage established by the reference standard. These comparisons indicate how many people were correctly classified as belonging to various stages of the disease, which allows us to calculate the test performance metrics of sensitivity, specificity, accuracy, and over-, and understaging. The selection of the reference standard is important in evaluating the true performance of an imaging modality for staging.

Comparators:
- Any direct comparisons of the imaging tests of interest
- Any direct comparisons of variations of any of the imaging tests of interest (e.g., contrast enhanced MRI vs. not enhanced MRI)

Outcomes:
- Test performance outcomes
  - Test performance (e.g., sensitivity, specificity, accuracy, over-, and understaging) against a reference standard test (pathologic examination, clinical followup, or intraoperative findings)
- Intermediate outcomes
  - Stage reclassification
  - Changes in therapeutic management
- Clinical outcomes
  - Overall mortality
  - Colorectal cancer–specific mortality
  - Quality of life and anxiety

- o Need for additional staging tests, including invasive procedures
- o Need for additional treatment, including surgery, radiotherapy, or chemotherapy
- o Resource use related to testing and treatment (when reported in the included studies)
- Adverse effects and harms
  - o Harms of testing per se (e.g., radiation exposure)
  - o Harms from test-directed treatments (e.g., overtreatment, undertreatment)

Timing:
- Primary staging
- Interim restaging
- Duration of followup will vary by outcome (e.g., from no followup for test performance measurements to many years for mortality)

Setting:
Any setting will be considered.

Conceptual Framework

An analytic framework illustrating the connections between the populations of interest, the staging modalities, and the outcomes is shown in Figure 1. Note the patient populations of interest are patients with newly diagnosed colorectal cancer or recurrent colorectal cancer. Populations that have completed treatment for colorectal cancer and are undergoing surveillance for recurrences are outside the scope of this report, as are asymptomatic individuals who are undergoing screening or individuals suspected of having cancer undergoing diagnostic workup. The use of imaging in diagnosing colorectal cancer is also outside the scope of this report.

The populations of interest enter the diagram at the left, undergo primary staging (Key Question 1), and then commence treatment. Some patients also undergo restaging after completing presurgical treatments such as chemotherapy (Key Question 2) and then proceed with treatment. Intermediate outcomes such as test performance and harms of testing can be measured immediately after performing the tests, but many of the relevant patient-oriented outcomes (such as mortality) can be measured only after completion of treatment. The point in the process at which each key question is most relevant is shown on the figure by the placement of the key question number (1 or 2) and subpart (e.g., a, b, c). The modifying factors affecting test performance in both the primary staging and restaging settings are shown in a separate box at the bottom of the figure.

Although not specified in the figure for simplicity, the four primary patient populations will be considered separately—patients with recurrent versus primary disease and primary staging versus interim restaging. If the data permitted it, additional groups were to be considered separately—rectal versus colon cancer, proximal colon versus distal colon cancer, and lower rectal versus middle rectal versus upper rectal cancer. However, the data permitted considering only rectal separately from colorectal cancer.

An important factor in selecting an imaging modality for staging is the availability of that modality. Although this factor will not be addressed formally via a key question, we collected and provide relevant information about the availability and accessibility of imaging modalities and information about current patterns of care. This information is presented in the discussion section to help place the evidence review findings in context.

Figure 1. Analytical framework of colorectal cancer staging review

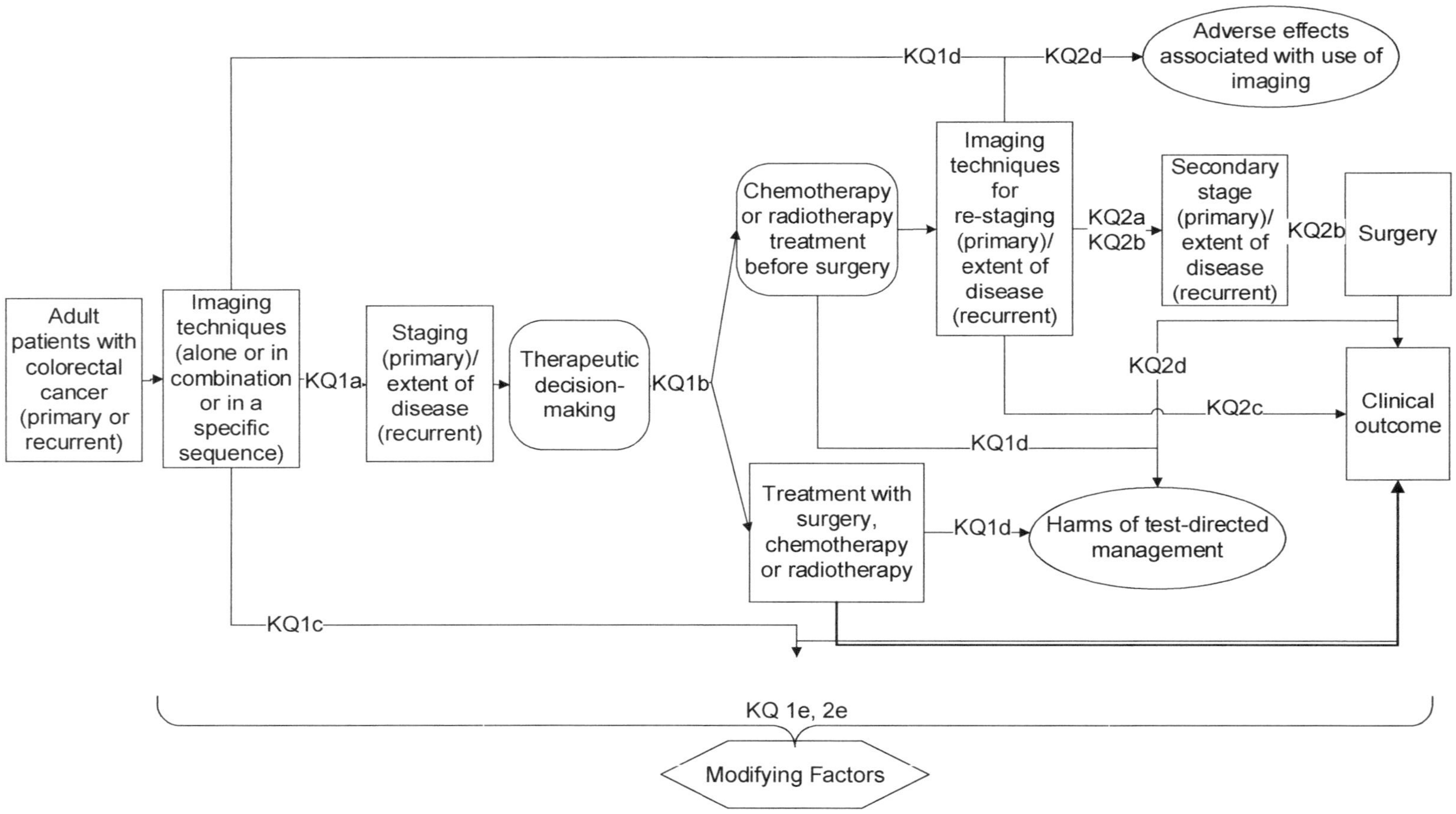

Organization of This Report

In the remaining three chapters of this report, we present the methods for this systematic review, the results for each key question, and a discussion of the findings. Within the Results chapter, we provide the results of the literature searches and screening procedures, then the results for Key Question 1. Findings for imaging studies of rectal cancer were reported separately, but those of colon cancer were reported in the literature only in mixed populations (rectal plus colon); consequently, we have presented findings specific to rectal cancer first, followed by results for colorectal cancer. We summarize the findings of previous systematic reviews on diagnostic accuracy of individual imaging modalities (ERUS, CT, MRI, and PET/CT) for staging of rectal and colorectal cancer before initial treatment, supplemented by an assessment of primary studies of PET/CT diagnostic accuracy for these indications. Following this, we present our assessment of primary studies comparing accuracy of one of these imaging modalities to another for TNM staging of rectal and colorectal cancer. We also present findings in terms of impact of the imaging results on therapeutic management. We then present reports of adverse events associated with the imaging techniques and finally, the patient, disease, and technical factors that affect the accuracy of the imaging studies. The results for Key Question 2, on restaging cancer in patients with primary and recurrent rectal and colorectal cancer after initial treatment, are presented in a similar order.

A list of acronyms and abbreviations is available following the list of references for this report. The Appendixes include Appendix A. Search Strategy, Appendix B. Excluded Studies, Appendix C. Evidence Tables and Appendix D. Analyses and Risk of Bias Assessments.

Methods

This section describes how the key questions were developed, how the literature was searched, how the included articles were selected, and how the data were analyzed. These methods follow those suggested in the ARHQ "Methods Guide for Effectiveness and Comparative Effectiveness Reviews" (available at www.effectivehealthcare.ahrq.gov/methodsguide.cfm).

Topic Refinement and Review Protocol

The topic was nominated in a public process. The Tufts Evidence-based Practice Center (EPC) recruited a panel of Key Informants (listed in the Acknowledgements section of the Front Matter) to provide input on the selection and refinement of the questions to be examined.

Upon AHRQ approval, the draft key questions were posted for public comment for four weeks on the AHRQ website. After receipt of public commentary, the SRC finalized the Key Questions and submitted them to AHRQ for approval. These Key Questions are presented in the Scope and Key Questions section of the Introduction.

Our EPC drafted a protocol and recruited a panel of content experts (the Technical Expert Panel, or TEP, listed in the Acknowledgements section of the Front Matter). Working in concert with AHRQ and the TEP, a plan for developing the evidence report was created. The protocol outlining the report's objectives, key questions, and methods was finalized and posted for public viewing. There were no deviations from the protocol during the review.

Individuals with broad expertise and perspectives were sought for the TEP. Divergent and conflicted opinions are common and perceived as healthy scientific discourse that results in a thoughtful, relevant systematic review. Therefore, in the end, study questions, design, and/or methodologic approaches do not necessarily represent the views of individual technical and content experts.

Literature Search Strategy

Search Strategy

Medical Librarians in the EPC Information Center performed literature searches following established systematic review protocols. We searched the following databases using controlled vocabulary and text words: EMBASE, MEDLINE, PubMed, and the Cochrane Library from 1980 through November 2013.

The following gray literature sources were searched using text words: ClinicalTrials.gov, Centers for Medicare & Medicaid (CMS) Medicare Coverage Database, ECRI Health Devices, Healthcare Standards, Internet, Medscape, National Guideline Clearinghouse™ (NGC), and the U.S. Food and Drug Administration (FDA).

The full search strategy is shown in Appendix A.

Inclusion and Exclusion Criteria

As suggested in the "Methods Guide for Comparative Effectiveness Reviews," we used inclusion criteria, listed below, in categories pertaining to publication type, study design, patient characteristics, test characteristics, and reported data.[8]

Publication criteria:

a. Full-length articles. The article must have been published as a full-length peer-reviewed study. Abstracts and meeting presentations were not included because they do not include sufficient details about experimental methods to permit an evaluation of study design and conduct, and they may also contain only a subset of measured outcomes.[66,67] In addition, it is not uncommon for abstracts that are published as part of conference proceedings to have inconsistencies when compared with the study's final publication or to describe studies that are never published as full articles.[68-72]

b. Redundancy. To avoid double-counting patients, in cases in which several reports of the same or overlapping groups of patients were available, only outcome data from the report with the largest number of patients were included. We included data from smaller studies when the smaller study reported data on an outcome that was not provided by the largest report or reported longer followup data for an outcome.

c. English language. Moher et al. have demonstrated that excluding non-English-language studies from meta-analyses has little impact on the conclusions drawn.[73] Juni et al. found that non-English studies were typically at higher risk of bias and that excluding them had little effect on effect-size estimates in the majority of meta-analyses they examined.[74] Although we recognize that in some situations exclusion of non-English studies could lead to bias, we believe that the few instances in which this may occur do not justify the time and cost typically necessary for translation of studies.

Study design criteria:

a. Single test performance. For questions about the performance of a single imaging test against a reference standard, we used a two-stage inclusion process. To avoid duplicating work, we first included only recent (2009 or later) high-quality systematic reviews. We included older reviews and primary studies only if the evidence from recent systematic reviews was insufficient to support an estimate of test performance for a particular imaging test (in this case, only PET/CT).

b. Comparative test performance. For questions about comparative test performance, we considered for inclusion studies of any design—randomized, cross-sectional, case-control, or cohort. Both retrospective and prospective studies were considered for inclusion, but retrospective studies must have used consecutive/all enrollment or enrollment of a random sample of participants. Studies must have directly compared two (or more) tests of interest and must have verified the results with a reference standard. The same reference standard must have been used to verify both (or all) tests.

c. Stage reclassification or clinical decision impact. For questions about stage reclassification or impact on clinician decisionmaking, cross-sectional, cohort, or prospective comparative (randomized or nonrandomized) studies were considered for inclusion.

d. Clinical outcomes. For questions about the impact of testing on patient-oriented clinical outcomes, comparative studies (randomized or nonrandomized) were considered for inclusion.

e. Harms. The adverse events and harms reported by any studies that addressed any of the other questions were used to address questions about harms and adverse events.

Additionally, we searched specifically for reports of harms and adverse events associated with the use of each specific imaging modality, such as radiation exposure and reactions to contrast agents. Any study design, including modeling, was acceptable for inclusion for questions about harms.

Patient criteria:

a. Type of patient. To be included, the study must have reported data obtained from groups of patients in which at least 85 percent were from one of the four patient populations of interest. These populations are: (1) patients with newly diagnosed colorectal disease undergoing primary staging, (2) patients with newly diagnosed colorectal disease undergoing interim restaging, (3) patients with newly diagnosed recurrent colorectal disease undergoing primary staging, and (4) patients with newly diagnosed recurrent colorectal disease undergoing interim restaging.

Although we have grouped all colon and rectal cancers together as "colorectal cancer" as an inclusion criterion, colon and rectal cancer are somewhat different diseases. Although we did not require that studies report only on rectal cancer or only on colon cancer for inclusion in the report, whenever possible (as permitted by the reported data) we analyzed the data for rectal and colon cancer separately; however, the data permitted only analyzing rectal separately from colorectal. The location of the rectal tumor—low, middle, or high—may also affect staging accuracy, so we had also planned, if possible, to analyze the data by subgroups of rectal tumor location. However, the nature of the reported data did not permit these analyses. Some evidence suggests that proximal and distal colon cancers may also be distinctly different conditions,[75] so we had planned to analyze data separately by proximal or distal subgroups, but none of the studies reported information separately for such subgroups.

b. Adults. Only studies of adult patients (older than 17 years of age) were considered for inclusion.

Test criteria:

a. Type of test. Only studies of the tests or comparisons of interest were considered for inclusion:
    i. Endoscopic rectal ultrasound (ERUS)
    ii. Magnetic resonance imaging (MRI)
    iii. Computed tomography (CT)
    iv. Positron emission tomography combined with computerized tomography PET/CT

b. Reference standards to assess test performance must have been one of the following:
    i. Histopathologic examination of tissue
    ii. Intraoperative findings
    iii. Clinical followup

c. Obsolete technology. In imaging technologies, there is constant innovation, research, and improvements in technology. Therefore, a need exists to identify and avoid obsolete technologies that have fallen out of routine clinical practice. Using a single cutoff date (for example, 2001) as a mechanism to eliminate obsolete technology is not thought to be appropriate. Instead, the TEP was consulted about which imaging technologies and variants of imaging technologies are now obsolete and not relevant to clinical practice. The imaging technologies that were determined to be obsolete (after discussion and consensus) for staging colorectal cancer are: transabdominal ultrasound, MRI using endorectal coils, nonmultidetector CT, CT arterial portography, CT angiography, CT colonography, and stand-alone PET. Likewise, experimental technology and prototypes were excluded on the grounds that there is currently insufficient evidence to evaluate their use; including them in this current review would serve no useful purpose. The TEP indicated that PET/MRI and PET/fused with CT colonography are considered to be experimental. MRI using ultrasmall paramagnetic iron oxide is also considered experimental.[28]

Data criteria:

a. The study must have reported data pertaining to one of the outcomes of interest (see the Key Questions section for a list).
b. We included data from time points and outcomes reported from groups of patients with at least 10 patients with the condition of interest who represented at least 50 percent of the patients originally enrolled in the study.

Study Selection

We screened the literature in duplicate using the database Distiller SR (Evidence Partners Incorporated, Ottawa, Canada). Literature search results were initially screened in duplicate for relevancy, and relevant abstracts were screened against the inclusion and exclusion criteria in duplicate. Studies that appeared from the abstract to meet the inclusion criteria were retrieved and screened again in duplicate against the inclusion and exclusion criteria.

Data Abstraction

Data were abstracted using the database Distiller SR. Data abstraction forms were constructed in Distiller, and the data were abstracted into these forms. Duplicate abstraction was used to ensure accuracy.

Abstracted elements include general study characteristics, patient characteristics, details of the imaging methodology, risk of bias items, and outcome data.

Individual Study Quality (Risk of Bias) Evaluation

For studies of test performance, we used an internal validity rating scale for diagnostic studies to assess the risk of bias of each individual study. This instrument is based on a modification of the QUADAS instrument with reference to empirical studies of design-related bias in diagnostic test studies.[76-78] Each question in the instrument addresses an aspect of study design or conduct that can help protect against bias, such as enrolling consecutive or a random sampling of patients or blinding image readers to a patient's clinical information. Each question can be answered "yes," "no," or "not reported," and each is phrased such that an answer of "yes" indicates that the study reported a protection against bias on that aspect. The instrument is shown in Appendix D.

Test performance studies were rated as low, medium, or high risk of bias. The rating was defined by selecting critical questions from the rating scale that must be answered "yes." The critical questions for these ratings for this review were selected after discussions with the TEP. For this topic, for a diagnostic study to be rated as low risk of bias, questions 1 and 3 (patient enrollment methods), question 6 (blinding of readers), and question 10 (avoided verification bias) must all be answered "yes," and at least six of the other questions must be answered "yes." The trial was rated at high risk of bias if all four critical questions were answered "no." The trial was rated at moderate risk of bias if it did not meet the criteria for low or high.

For controlled studies, we used an internal validity rating scale for comparative studies to assess each study's risk of bias. ECRI Institute developed this instrument[79] with reference to empirical studies of the impact of study design on bias in comparative studies and is consistent with the guidance in the "Methods Guide for Comparative Effectiveness Reviews."[80] Each question in the instrument addresses an aspect of study design or conduct that can help protect against bias, such as randomization of group assignment, or blinding outcome assessors to patient group assignment. Each question can be answered "yes," "no," or "not reported," and each is phrased such that an answer of "yes" indicates that the study reported a protection against bias on that aspect. The instrument is shown in Appendix D.

Controlled studies were rated as low, medium, or high risk of bias. The rating is defined by selecting critical questions from the rating scale that must be answered "yes." The critical questions for these ratings for this review were selected after discussions with the TEP. For this topic, for a controlled/comparative study to be rated as low risk of bias, questions 1, 2, and 4 (appropriately randomized or used methods to enhance group comparability) and questions 6 and 7 (group comparability) must all be answered "yes," and at least 10 of the other questions must be answered "yes." The trial was rated at high risk of bias if all five critical questions were answered "no." The trial was rated at moderate risk of bias if it did not meet the criteria for low or high.

As the "Methods Guide for Comparative Effectiveness Reviews" suggests, the quality of systematic reviews used to address Key Questions 1a and 2a was assessed with a modified AMSTAR instrument.[6] The instrument is shown in Appendix C.

Systematic reviews were rated as either high quality or not. The rating was defined by selecting critical questions from the rating scale that must be answered "yes." The critical questions for these ratings for this review were selected after discussions with the TEP. For this topic, for a systematic review to be rated as high quality, questions 2 and 2a (search methods), 4 and 4a (study inclusion), 7, 7a, and 7b (rating of study quality and strength of evidence), 8 (methods of analysis) and 10 (conflicts of interest) all need to be answered "yes." Only high-quality systematic reviews were included to address Key Questions 1a and 2a.

Data Analysis and Synthesis

For questions addressing individual test performance (accuracy), we have drawn evidence from prior systematic reviews. As recommended by the "Methods Guide," we have summarized all relevant high-quality reviews.[6]

For comparative questions, we synthesized the evidence from the primary studies themselves. We performed meta-analysis as appropriate and possible. Decisions about whether meta-analysis was appropriate were based on the judged clinical homogeneity of the different study populations, imaging and treatment protocols, and outcomes. . In order to avoid the possibility of outcome reporting bias, if fewer than 75% of the studies in an available evidence base could be combined in a quantitative meta-analysis (for any reason(s)), we refrained from performing a quantitative analysis. In cases in which meta-analysis was not possible (because of limitations of reported data) or was judged to be inappropriate, the data were synthesized using a descriptive approach.

For studies of clinical outcomes and analyses of accuracy, we computed effect sizes (odds ratios for paired data of error) and measures of variance using standard methods, and performed DerSimonian and Laird random-effects meta-analysis using Comprehensive Meta-Analysis (CMA) software (Biostat, Inc., Englewood, NJ). . Becasue studies did not report the correlations among tests, we assumed a correlation of 0.5, and performed sensitivity analyses using correlations of 0.1 and 0.9.

We next provide a worked example of how we calculated the accuracy data. Box 1 below shows the hypothetical results from a single study. Each patient was assigned a T stage (1, 2, 3 or 4) by both CT and ERUS, and the correct stage for each patient was determined by the reference standard. The shaded cells indicate patients who have been correctly staged.

Box 1. Sample accuracy data

CT	pT1	pT2	pT3	pT4	ERUS	pT1	pT2	pT3	pT4
T1	0	0	0	0	T1	7	2	0	0
T2	7	16	7	0	T2	0	21	2	0
T3	0	9	22	3	T3	0	2	27	2
T4	0	0	4	10	T4	0	0	2	11

To calculate accuracy (actually the odds ratio of incorrectly staging), the number of correct cases are added and subtracted from the total and then divided by the total:
- Odds of incorrect stage for CT=((78–48)/78)/((78–30)/78)=0.385/0.615=0.625
- Odds of incorrect stage for ERUS=((76–66)/76)/((76–10)/76)=0.132/0.868=0.152
- Odds ratio of incorrect stageCT vs. ERUS=0.625/0.152=4.125

If the odds ratio is 1.0 or close to 1.0, there is no apparent difference between the two modalities in accuracy; for this example, if the result is greater than one, ERUS (the denominator) is more accurate.

To calculate the odds ratio of understaging, note that the cells above the shaded cells represent understaged patients, and they are the only ones treated as errors for the purpose of an understaging analysis:
- Odds of understaging by CT=((78–68)/78)/((78-10)/78)=0.128/0.872=0.147
- Odds of understaging by ERUS=((76–70)/76)/((76–6)/76)=0.079/0.921=0.086
- Odds ratio of understaging for CT vs. ERUS=0.147/0.086=1.716

To calculate odds ratio of overstaging, the calculations are similar to those understaging, above, except the only ones treated as errors are those below the shaded cells.

Because the same patients underwent both tests being compared, and studies did not report the correlations among tests, we assumed a correlation of 0.5, and performed sensitivity analyses using correlations of 0.1 and 0.9.

For studies of test performance, we meta-analyzed the data reported by the studies using a bivariate random-effects binomial regression model as described by Harbord et al.[10] All such analyses were computed by the STATA 13.0 statistical software package (StataCorp. LP, College Station, TX) using the metandi command.[11] In cases in which a binomial-bivariate normal regression model could not be fit due to insufficient number of studies (n<4), we meta-analyzed the diagnostic data using a random-effects model and the software package Meta-Disc (freeware developed by the Unit of Clinical Biostatistics, Ramón y Cajal Hospital, Madrid, Spain).[12]

Wherever possible, we have performed calculations of standard diagnostic test characteristics (sensitivity, specificity) and calculations of accuracy, under- and over-staging. If the two different approaches to analysis produced different conclusions about which test is to be preferred for that situation, the data were categorized as inconsistent/ heterogeneous.

Subgroup analysis has been used to explore possible causes of heterogeneity. Covariates include population descriptors, tumor site and type, country and setting of care, variations in imaging technology, and publication date.

Strength of Evidence Grading

We used a formal grading system that conforms with the "Methods Guide for Comparative Effectiveness Reviews" recommendations on grading the strength of evidence.[7-9]

The overall strength of evidence supporting each major conclusion was graded as high, moderate, low, or insufficient. The grade was developed by considering four important domains: study limitations, consistency of findings, precision of the results, and directness of the evidence. We assessed the risk of bias of each individual study (see section "Assessing Quality of Individual Studies") for each outcome and used the aggregate risk of bias to describe the study limitations of the entire evidence base for the comparison and outcome (generally, the median risk of bias across the evidence base—for example, if five studies are rated as low risk of bias and two are rated as moderate risk of bias, the study limitations of the entire evidence base for that outcome would be rated as low). Consistency of the evidence was assessed by considering study populations, imaging and treatment protocols, study designs and outcomes, in addition to statistical heterogeneity. We rated the consistency of conclusions supported by random effects meta-analyses with the statistic I^2.[81,82] Data sets that are found to have an I^2 of less than 50 percent were rated as being consistent; 50 percent or greater were rated as being inconsistent; and data sets for which I^2 could not be calculated (e.g., a single study) were rated as consistency unknown. For qualitative comparisons, we rated conclusions as consistent if the effect sizes were all in the same direction. We used the width of the 95 percent confidence intervals around the summary effect sizes to evaluate the precision of the evidence. If the study directly addressed a key question, the evidence was rated as direct.

We used the following process to grade the evidence: the base grade was chosen based on the study limitations for the evidence base. If the level of study limitations was judged to be low, the grade started at highat high; if the study limitations were at a medium level, the grade started at moderate; and if the level of study limitations was high, the grade started at low. If the evidence base consisted of only one study, it was automatically rated as insufficient. If the evidence was not consistent, it was downgraded one step; if it was not precise (or if precision could not be determined), it was downgraded by one step; and if not direct, it also was downgraded by one step. We intended to use an additional criterion (order of magnitude of effect); if the effect was judged to be extremely large, we would upgrade one step; however, this situation did not occur.

Publication bias was addressed by inspection of funnel plots supplemented with information from the included systematic reviews. We also looked for evidence that earlier publications were more likely to report positive findings.

We did not grade the strength of evidence from published systematic reviews, but as described previously, we assessed their quality using the modified AMSTAR instrument.

Applicability

The applicability of the evidence involves four key aspects: patients, tests or interventions, comparisons and settings.[83] After discussions with the TEP, we concluded that age and sex of patients is unlikely to affect the accuracy of staging, but other patient characteristics, such as race, obesity, genetic syndromes predisposing to colorectal cancer, and enrollment of populations with high rates of comorbid conditions, could affect the applicability of study findings, particularly with regard to patient-oriented outcomes. After consulting with the TEP, we addressed test and interventions and comparisons by excluding obsolete and experimental imaging tests from the report.

Peer Review and Public Commentary

Peer reviewers were invited to provide written comments on the draft based on their clinical, content, or methodologic expertise. AHRQ and an EPC Associate Editor also provided comments. The draft report was posted on the AHRQ Web site for 4 weeks to elicit public comment. Reviewer comments on the preliminary draft were considered by the EPC in preparing the final report. Peer reviewers do not participate in writing or editing the final report or other products. The synthesis of the scientific literature presented in the final report does not necessarily represent the views of individual reviewers. The dispositions of the peer-review and public comments are documented and will be published 3 months after the publication of the Evidence Report.

Potential reviewers must disclose any financial conflicts of interest greater than $10,000 and any other relevant business or professional conflicts of interest. Invited peer reviewers may not have any financial conflict of interest greater than $10,000. Peer reviewers who disclose potential business or professional conflicts of interest may submit comments on draft reports through the public comment mechanism.

Results

Introduction

In this chapter, we describe the evidence in terms of literature search results and screening procedures. We then present the results for each key question. Findings for imaging studies of rectal cancer were often reported separately, but those of colon cancer were not reported separately in any studies that met the inclusion criteria; they were reported only in the included studies mixed with rectal cancer cases, as "colorectal" cancer; consequently, we have presented findings for rectal cancer first, followed by results for colorectal cancer. Under Key Question 1, we summarize the findings of previous systematic reviews on diagnostic accuracy of individual imaging modalities (endoscopic rectal ultrasound [ERUS], computed tomography [CT], magnetic resonance imaging [MRI], and positron emission tomography/computed tomography [PET/CT]) for staging rectal and colorectal cancer before initial treatment, supplemented by an assessment of primary studies of PET/CT diagnostic accuracy for these indications. Following this, we present our assessment of primary studies comparing accuracy of one imaging modality to another for TNM staging of rectal and colorectal cancer. These sections are organized by the type of staging under consideration. We also present results of studies of the impact of imaging on therapeutic management. We then present reports of adverse events associated with the imaging techniques and the patient, disease, and technical factors that affect the accuracy of the imaging studies. The results for Key Question 2, on restaging cancer in patients with primary and recurrent rectal and colorectal cancer after initial treatment, are presented in a similar fashion.

A list of acronyms and abbreviations is available following the list of references for this report. The Appendixes include Appendix A. Search Strategy, Appendix B. Excluded Studies, Appendix C. Evidence Tables and Appendix D. Analyses and Risk of Bias Assessments.

Results of Literature Searches

The study selection process is summarized in Figure 2. The literature searches identified 4,683 citations. After review of the abstracts of these articles in duplicate, 4,473 were excluded. The most common reason for exclusion was lack of relevancy to the key questions (off topic). Some of the excluded narrative reviews and patterns of care articles were used to inform the background section and the patterns of care section. In all, 210 articles were retrieved in full, 31 of which were thought to be systematic reviews and were screened against the systematic review inclusion criteria, and 179 that were thought to be clinical studies and were screened against the clinical study inclusion criteria. See the "Methods" chapter for the inclusion criteria. After screening the articles in duplicate, 8 systematic reviews and 65 primary clinical studies were included. See Appendix B for a list of the excluded studies.

Figure 2. Study flow diagram

```
┌─────────────────────────────────────┐
│ 4,683 Citations identified by       │
│        literature searches          │
└─────────────────────────────────────┘
              │
              ▼
         ╱╲                         ┌──────────────────────────────────────┐
        ╱  ╲                        │    4,473 Citations excluded:         │
       ╱ Abs-╲                      │  3,273  Off topic                    │
      ╱tracts ╲ ─────────────────▶ │  1,011  Narrative reviews            │
      ╲screened╱                    │     58  Animal study                 │
       ╲      ╱                     │     58  Not in English               │
        ╲    ╱                      │     40  Clinical practice guideline  │
         ╲╱                         │     28  Patterns of care             │
          │                         │      5  Meeting abstracts            │
          ▼                         └──────────────────────────────────────┘
┌─────────────────────────────────────┐
│    210 Articles retrieved:          │   ┌────────────────────────────────────────┐
│       31 systematic reviews         │   │  23 Systematic reviews excluded:       │
│       179 primary studies           │   │  9  Published before 2009              │
└─────────────────────────────────────┘   │  6  Not a systematic review            │
              │                           │  5  Not high-quality                   │
              ▼                           │  1  Not colorectal cancer              │
          ╱╲                              │  1  No outcomes of interest            │
         ╱  ╲                             │  1  Patients not diagnosed with cancer │
        ╱    ╲                            │     before enrollment                  │
       ╱ Arti-╲                           │   114 Primary articles excluded:       │
      ╱ cles   ╲ ──────────────────────▶ │  16 None of the test comparisons of   │
      ╲reviewed╱                          │     interest                           │
       ╲      ╱                           │  19 Mixed types of patients            │
        ╲    ╱                            │  15 Not a clinical study               │
         ╲╱                               │  10 Experimental technology            │
          │                               │   9 Obsolete technology                │
          ▼                               │   7 Off topic                          │
┌─────────────────────────────────────┐   │   7 Not in English                     │
│      8 Systematic reviews           │   │   6 Not about colorectal cancer        │
│      65 Clinical studies            │   │   6 More than 50% of patients lost     │
└─────────────────────────────────────┘   │   6 Cancer not diagnosed in patients   │
                                          │     before enrollment                  │
                                          │   3 None of the outcomes of interest   │
                                          │   3 Retrospective study that did not   │
                                          │     enroll all or consecutive patients │
                                          │   4 No reference standard              │
                                          │   1 Duplicate report of same patients  │
                                          │   1 Too few patients                   │
                                          │   1 Different reference standards for  │
                                          │     different groups of patients       │
                                          └────────────────────────────────────────┘
```

Test Performance of Imaging Modalities for Pretreatment Staging

Key Question 1. What is the comparative effectiveness of imaging techniques for pretreatment cancer staging in patients with primary and recurrent colorectal cancer?

Key Question 1a. What is the test performance of the imaging techniques used (singly, in combination, or in a specific sequence) to stage colorectal cancer compared with a reference standard?

Key Points

We addressed Key Question 1a using systematic reviews supplemented by assessment of primary studies if insufficient evidence from systematic reviews was available. Seven recent (2009 or later) high-quality systematic reviews met the inclusion criteria for this question (Table 6) and analyzed accuracy of ERUS, MRI, CT, and PET/CT for staging colorectal cancer. There was insufficient information from systematic reviews for PET/CT, so primary studies were used to assess the test performance of PET/CT.

Table 6. Included systematic reviews addressing accuracy of ERUS, MRI, CT, or PET/CT

Study	Modalities Studied	Condition	Databases Searched	Dates Searched	Inclusion Criteria	Primary Method of Analysis	Number of Articles	Number of Patients	Study Quality
Gall et al. 2013[84]	ERUS (mini-probe only)	Colorectal	MEDLINE, EMBASE, Cochrane	Through January 2013	Studies of mini-probe ERUS for staging of colon cancer or mixed colorectal that used histopathology as the reference standard and staged using the TNM system.	Bivariate and hierarchical summary receiver operating characteristics model	10 total; 5 included patients with colon cancer only, 5 had mixed colorectal populations	642 total; 210 colon cancer	All studies had 8 or more of the 14 QUADAS items

Table 6. Included systematic reviews addressing accuracy of ERUS, MRI, CT, or PET/CT (continued)

Study	Modalities Studied	Condition	Databases Searched	Dates Searched	Inclusion Criteria	Primary Method of Analysis	Number of Articles	Number of Patients	Study Quality
Puli et al. 2009[85]	ERUS	Rectal cancer	MEDLINE, PubMed, EMBASE, CINAHL, Cochrane, DARE, Healthstar	1966 to January 2008	Full-length published studies of rectal cancer N staging confirmed by surgical histology that reported sufficient data to construct 2x2 tables	Random-effects or fixed-effects pooling of sensitivity/specificity separately	35	2,732	All of the studies fulfilled 4 to 5 out of the 14 QUADAS items
Puli et al. 2009[14]	ERUS	Rectal cancer	MEDLINE, PubMed, EMBASE, CINAHL, Cochrane, DARE, Healthstar	1980 to January 2008	Full-length published studies of T staging rectal cancer with endoscopic ultrasound using surgical histology as the reference standard and sufficient data to construct 2x2 tables	Random-effects or fixed-effects pooling of sensitivity/specificity separately	42	5,039	All of the studies fulfilled 4 to 5 out of the 14 QUADAS items

Table 6. Included systematic reviews addressing accuracy of ERUS, MRI, CT, or PET/CT (continued)

Study	Modalities Studied	Condition	Databases Searched	Dates Searched	Inclusion Criteria	Primary Method of Analysis	Number of Articles	Number of Patients	Study Quality
Al-Sukhni et al. 2012[86]	MRI	Rectal cancer	MEDLINE, EMBASE, Cochrane	January 2000 to March 2011	English-language original published reports of MRI using a phase-array coil, histopathology as the reference standard, and sufficient data reported to construct 2x2 tables	Bivariate random-effects model and hierarchical summary receiver operating characteristics model	19 studies for T stage, 12 studies for N stage, 10 studies for CRM	1,986 patients for T stage, 1,249 patients for N stage, 986 patients for CRM	62% of the studies had 10 or more of the 13 modified QUADAS items
Dighe et al. 2010[16]	CT	Colon cancer primarily, a few studies mixed colorectal	MEDLINE, EMBASE, Cochrane	Through March 5, 2009	Published preoperative N staging using histopathology as the reference standard and sufficient data reported to calculate TP, TN, FP, and FN	Bivariate random-effects model	19 total; 17 reported on T stage, 15 on N stage	907 total, 784 T stage, 674 N stage	53% of studies scored 12 or higher on the QUADAS items

Table 6. Included systematic reviews addressing accuracy of ERUS, MRI, CT, or PET/CT (continued)

Study	Modalities Studied	Condition	Databases Searched	Dates Searched	Inclusion Criteria	Primary Method of Analysis	Number of Articles	Number of Patients	Study Quality
Lu et al. 2012[87]	PET/CT, PET	Colorectal cancer	MEDLINE, PubMed, EMBASE	Through February 2012	Full-length published articles of nodal staging by PET or PET/CT in patients with colorectal cancer with sufficient data reported to derive 2x2 tables	Random-effects or fixed-effects pooling of sensitivity/specificity separately	8 PET, 2 PET/CT	83 PET/CT, 326 PET	On the Cochrane Diagnostic Tests tool, the mean quality score was 59.2%, Range: 33% to 83%

Table 6. Included systematic reviews addressing accuracy of ERUS, MRI, CT, or PET/CT (continued)

Study	Modalities Studied	Condition	Databases Searched	Dates Searched	Inclusion Criteria	Primary Method of Analysis	Number of Articles	Number of Patients	Study Quality
Niekel et al. 2010[15]	CT, MRI, PET/CT	Colorectal liver metastases	MEDLINE, EMBASE, Cochrane, CINAHL, Web of Science	January 1990 to January 2010	Prospective full-length, published articles with at least 10 patients with histopathologically proven colorectal cancer undergoing evaluation for liver metastases that reported sufficient data to allow calculation of sensitivity and specificity	Random-effects or fixed-effects pooling of sensitivity/specificity separately	25 CT, 18 MRI, 5 PET/CT	3,391	65% of the studies had 6 or more of the 10 modified QUADAS items

CINAHL=Cumulative Index to Nursing and Allied Health Literature; CRM=circumferential resection margin; DARE=Database of Reviews of Effectiveness; ERUS=endorectal ultrasound; FN=false negative; FP=false positive; MRI=magnetic resonance imaging; N=nodal stage; PET=positron emission tomography; PET/CT=positron emission tomography/computed tomography; QUADAS=quality assessment tool for diagnostic accuracy studies; T=tumor stage; TN=true negative; TP=true positive.

Detailed Synthesis

Endoscopic Rectal Ultrasound

One group (Puli et al.) conducted two systematic reviews of the accuracy of ERUS for staging rectal cancer; one of the reviews covered nodal (N) staging; the other covered tumor (T) staging. Another group conducted a systematic review of colorectal staging, but using a particular type of probe (mini-probe) only. The results are summarized in Table 7.

Table 7. Results from included systematic reviews for endoscopic rectal ultrasound

Study	Included Articles	Number of Patients	Primary Results	Author's Conclusion
Gall et al. 2013[84]	10	642	T1: sensitivity 91% (95% CI, 76 to 97%), specificity 98% (95% CI, 97 to 99); T2 sensitivity 78% (95% CI, 62 to 88), specificity 94% (95% CI, 91 to 96); T3/T4: sensitivity 97% (95% CI, 91 to 99), specificity 90% (95% CI 85 to 94); N: sensitivity 63% (95% CI 47 to 77), specificity 82% (95% CI 73 to 89).	Mini-probe ERUS is effective in staging colorectal cancer.
Puli et al. 2009[85]	35	2,732	ERUS for N staging: Sensitivity of 73.2% (95% CI, 70.6 to 75.6); Specificity 75.8% (95% CI, 73.5 to 78.0), +LR 2.84 (95% CI, 2.16 to 3.72), -LR 0.42 (95% CI, 0.33 to 0.52)	ERUS is an important and accurate diagnostic tool for evaluating nodal metastasis of rectal cancers. This meta-analysis shows that the sensitivity and specificity of ERUS is moderate.
Puli et al. 2009[14]	42	5,039	ERUS for T1: Sensitivity 87.8% (95% CI, 85.3 to 90.0), Specificity 98.3% (95% CI, 97.8 to 98.7), +LR 44.0 (95% CI, 22.7 to 85.5), -LR 0.16 (95% CI, 0.13 to 0.23)	As a result of the demonstrated sensitivity and specificity, ERUS should be the investigation of choice to T stage rectal cancers. The sensitivity of ERUS is higher for advanced disease than for early disease.
			ERUS for T2: Sensitivity 80.5% (95% CI, 77.9 to 82.9), Specificity 95.6% (95% CI, 94.9 to 96.3), +LR 17.3 (95% CI, 11.9 to 24.9), -LR 0.22 (95% CI, 0.17 to 0.29)	
			ERUS for T3: Sensitivity 96.4% (95% CI, 95.4 to 97.2), Specificity 90.6% (95% CI, 89.5 to 91.7), +LR 8.9 (95% CI, 6.8 to 11.8), -LR 0.06 (95% CI, 0.04 to 0.09)	
			ERUS for T4: Sensitivity 95.4% (95% CI, 92.4 to 97.5), Specificity 98.3% (95% CI, 97.8 to 98.7), +LR 37.6 (95% CI, 19.9 to 71.0), -LR 0.14 (95% CI, 0.09 to 0.23)	

CI=Confidence interval; ERUS=endoscopic rectal ultrasound; +LR=positive likelihood ratio; -LR=negative likelihood ratio; N=nodal stage; T=tumor stage.

Publication Bias

Puli et al. concluded that there was no evidence of publication bias in 2009; however, a systematic review published in 2005 (thus, not included to address the key questions) concluded that "the performance of EUS [endoscopic ultrasound] in staging rectal cancer may be overestimated in the literature due to publication bias."[13] The review included 41 studies published between 1985 and 2003. The author, Harewood, performed visual analyses of funnel diagrams and other plots, demonstrating that there appeared to be few smaller studies that found lower accuracy rates and that the reported accuracy appeared to be declining over time. Studies published in the surgical literature reported higher accuracies than studies published in other types of journals.[13] Declining accuracy over time and non-random patterns of accuracy in different types of journals both suggest the presence of publication and/or reporting bias.

Puli et al. also analyzed the reported accuracy of ERUS over time and found that the reported accuracy had declined significantly from the 1980s through 2000 and had stabilized or only declined slightly since.[14] Gall et al. did not assess the possibility of publication bias.[84]

Computed Tomography

Two groups published systematic reviews of the use of T for staging colorectal cancer; their results are summarized in Table 8.

Table 8. Results from included systematic reviews for computed tomography

Study	Included Articles	Number of Patients	Primary Results	Author's Conclusion
Niekel et al. 2010[15]	25 CT, 18 MRI, 5 PET/CT	3,391	Sensitivity of CT for liver metastasis: 83.6%	The sensitivity of CT was lower than either MRI or PET imaging.
Dighe et al. 2010[16]	19 total; 17 reported on T stage, 15 on N stage	907 total, 784 T stage, 674 N stage	CT T1/T2 differentiate from T3/T4 sensitivity 86% (95% CI, 78 to 92%), specificity 78% (95% CI, 71 to 84%)	Preoperative staging CT accurately distinguishes between tumors confined to the bowel wall and those invading beyond the MP; however, it is significantly poorer at identifying nodal status. MDCT provides the best results.
			CT T3 from T4 sensitivity 92% (95% CI, 87% to 95%), specificity 81% (95% CI, 70 to 89%)	
			CT N stage sensitivity 70% (95% CI, 59% to 80%), specificity 78% (95% CI, 66 to 86%)	

CI=Confidence interval; CT=computed tomography; MDCT=multidetector computed tomography; MP=muscularis propria; MRI=magnetic resonance imaging; N=nodal stage; PET/CT=positron emission tomography/computed tomography; T=tumor stage.

Publication Bias

Niekel et al. reported no evidence of publication bias for distant metastasis (M) staging by CT, but Dighe et al. reported that for N staging with CT there was evidence that smaller studies were reporting higher accuracies (suggesting publication bias) and that there was a nonsignificant trend showing the same result for T staging.[16]

Magnetic Resonance Imaging

Two groups reported on the accuracy of MRI, one for staging colorectal cancer (Niekel et al.) and the other for rectal cancer (Al-Sukhni et al.), summarized in Table 9.

Table 9. Results from included systematic reviews for MRI

Study	Included Articles	Number of Patients	Primary Results	Author's Conclusion
Al-Sukhni et al. 2012[86]	19 studies for T stage, 12 studies for N stage, 10 studies for CRM	1,986 patients for T stage, 1,249 patients for N stage, 986 patients for CRM	MRI for N: sensitivity 77% (95% CI, 69% to 84), specificity 71% (95% CI, 59% to 81%) MRI for T: sensitivity 87% (95% CI, 81% to 92%), specificity 75% (95% CI, 68% to 80%) MRI for CRM: sensitivity 77% (95% CI, 57 to 90), specificity 94% (95% CI, 88 to 97)	"MRI has good accuracy for both CRM and T category and should be considered for preoperative rectal cancer staging. In contrast, lymph node assessment is poor on MRI."
Niekel et al. 2010[15]	25 CT, 18 MRI, 5 PET/CT	3,391	Sensitivity of MRI for liver metastasis: 88.2%	"MRI imaging is the preferred first-line modality for evaluating colorectal liver metastases in patients who have not had earlier therapy."

CI=confidence interval; CRM=circumferential resection margin; MRI=magnetic resonance imaging; N=nodal stage; PET/CT=positron emission tomography/computed tomography; T=tumor stage.

Publication Bias

Niekel et al. reported there was no evidence of publication bias in the MRI staging literature.[15]

Positron Emission Tomography/Computed Tomography

One group (Lu et al.) published a systematic review on the accuracy of PET/CT for staging colorectal cancer, summarized in Table 10; however, they pooled data from eight studies of stand-alone PET with two studies of PET/CT. Another group (Niekel et al.) also published a systematic review on PET/CT, but concluded there was insufficient data.

Table 10. Results from included systematic reviews of PET/CT

Study	Included Articles	Number of Patients	Primary Results	Author's Conclusion
Lu et al. 2012[87]	8 PET, 2 PET/CT	83 PET/CT, 326 PET	The sensitivity of PET for detecting involved lymph nodes was 42.9% (95% CI, 36.0 to 50.0%); the specificity was 87.9% (95% CI, 82.6 to 92.0).	There is no solid evidence to support the routine clinical application of PET (PET/CT) in the pretherapeutic evaluation of lymph node status in patients with colorectal cancer.
Niekel et al. 2010[15]	25 CT, 18 MRI, 5 PET/CT	3,391	Sensitivity of PET/CT for liver metastasis: data were too limited.	The role of PET/CT is unclear because of the small number of studies.

CI=Confidence interval; CT=computed tomography; MRI=magnetic resonance imaging; PET=positron emission tomography; PET/CT=positron emission tomography/computed tomography.

Because there were insufficient recent (2009 or later) high-quality systematic reviews on PET/CT, we searched for high-quality, older systematic reviews but did not identify any that met the inclusion criteria. We therefore examined the studies of PET/CT included in this report to address the comparative questions; these results are summarized in Table 11.

Table 11. Results from included primary studies for PET/CT

Study	Number of Patients	Primary Results
Kim et al. 2011[88]	30 primary rectal	Rectal N staging: sensitivity 61%, specificity 83%
Uchiyama et al. 2012[89]	77 colorectal	Colorectal T staging: accuracy 95.0% Colorectal N staging: sensitivity 34.3%, specificity 100% Colorectal M staging: sensitivity 93.8%
Ramos et al. 2011[19]	70 colorectal	Colorectal M staging: sensitivity 72% (per lesion basis)
Orlacchio et al. 2009[90]	467 colorectal	Colorectal M staging: sensitivity 97.9%, specificity 97.7%
Lubezky et al. 2007[91]	27 colorectal	Colorectal M staging: sensitivity 93.3%

M=Distant metastasis stage; N=nodal stage; PET/CT=positron emission tomography/computed tomography; T=tumor stage.

Publication Bias

Neither systematic review on PET/CT evaluated the possibility of publication bias.

Comparative Test Performance of Imaging Modalities for Pretreatment Staging

Key Points

- ERUS is more accurate (odds ratio [OR]=0.36; 95% CI, 0.24 to 0.54), less likely to understage (OR=0.63; 95% CI, 0.44 to 0.89), and less likely to overstage (OR=0.47; 95% CI, 0.28 to 0.80) rectal cancer than CT in the preoperative T staging setting. Strength of evidence is low.
- There is no significant difference in accuracy between MRI and ERUS or between MRI and CT for preoperative rectal T staging. Strength of evidence is low.
- There is no significant difference in accuracy across CT, MRI, or ERUS for preoperative rectal N staging. MRI is less likely than CT to overstage (OR=0.498, 95% CI, 0.308 to 0.806). Strength of evidence is low.
- MRI is superior to CT in detecting colorectal liver metastases in the preoperative setting (OR=1.334; 95% CI, 1.012 to 1.761). Strength of evidence is moderate.
- The evidence was insufficient for drawing conclusions about the accuracy of PET/CT compared to either MRI or CT for rectal T, N, or M staging.

Detailed Synthesis

Preoperative Rectal Tumor Staging

We identified 23 studies of preoperative rectal T staging (summarized in Table 12). Six studies compared MRI with ERUS, 13 compared CT with ERUS, three compared MRI with CT, and one study compared CT, MRI, and ERUS.

Table 12. Preoperative rectal T staging

Study	Compares	Number of Patients	Design	Risk of Bias
Barbaro et al. 1995[92]	CT, MRI, ERUS	13	Cohort	Moderate
Yimei et al. 2012[93]	MRI to ERUS	129	Cohort	Moderate
Halefoglu et al. 2008[94]	MRI to ERUS	34	Cohort	Low
Bianchi et al. 2005[95]	MRI to ERUS	49	Cohort	Moderate
Starck et al. 1995[96]	MRI to ERUS	35	Prospective cohort	Moderate
Thaler et al. 1994[97]	MRI to ERUS	34	Prospective cohort	Low
Waizer et al. 1991[98]	MRI to ERUS	13	Prospective cohort	Moderate
Ju et al. 2009[99]	CT to ERUS	78	Cohort	Moderate
Kim et al. 1999[100]	CT to ERUS	89	Cohort	Moderate
Osti et al. 1997[101]	CT to ERUS	63	Cohort	Moderate
Ramana et al. 1997[102]	CT to ERUS	10	Prospective cohort	Moderate
Goldman et al. 1991[103]	CT to ERUS	29	Prospective cohort	Moderate
Pappalardo et al. 1990[104]	CT to ERUS	14	Prospective cohort	Moderate
Rotte et al. 1989[105]	CT to ERUS	25	Cohort	Moderate
Waizer et al. 1989[106]	CT to ERUS	58	Prospective cohort	Moderate
Beynon et al. 1986[107]	CT to ERUS	44	Prospective cohort	Moderate
Kramann and Hildebrandt 1986[108]	CT to ERUS	29	Cohort	Moderate
Rifkin and Wechsler 1986[109]	CT to ERUS	79	Prospective cohort	Moderate
Rifkin, McGlynn, and Marks 1986[110]	CT to ERUS	54	Prospective cohort	Moderate
Romano et al. 1985[111]	CT to ERUS	23	Cohort	Moderate
Matsuoka et al. 2003[112]	MRI to CT	21	Prospective cohort	Moderate
Guinet et al. 1990[113]	MRI to CT	19	Cohort	Moderate
Hodgman et al. 1986[114]	MRI to CT	30	Cohort	Moderate

CT=Computed tomography; ERUS=endorectal ultrasound; MRI=magnetic resonance imaging.

The data reported by the six studies of MRI versus ERUS for rectal T staging are shown in Appendix C. The diagnostic test characteristics reported by the five studies that reported diagnostic test characteristics are shown below, in Figure 3. We pooled the reported diagnostic data in a binomial-bivariate model of the diagnostic accuracy of distinguishing between T1/T2 and T3/T4 stages, and we also pooled the accuracy, over-, and understaging data in random-effects models. The full bivariate model and summary receiver operating characteristic (HSROC) curves are shown in Appendix D. The complete results of the random-effects models are reported in Appendix D and are summarized below, in Table 13. All of our analyses indicated that there was no significant difference between the MRI and ERUS. The level of study limitations was medium, and the data were consistent and direct but not very precise (wide confidence intervals); therefore, the strength of evidence is low.

The data reported by the 13 studies of CT versus ERUS for rectal T staging are shown in Appendix C. Because many of the studies reported insufficient data to calculate sensitivity and specificity, we pooled only the accuracy, over-, and understaging data in random-effects models. The full results of the analyses are shown in Appendix D and are shown graphically below in Figure 4 and Figure 5. The results are summarized below, in Table 13. ERUS was statistically significantly more accurate than CT and was statistically significantly less likely to over- or understage rectal cancer than CT. The level of study limitations was medium, and the data were consistent and direct but not precise (wide confidence intervals); although the effect size was large it was not extremely large; therefore, the strength of evidence is low.

The data reported by the three studies of MRI versus CT are shown in Appendix C. The oldest study, Hodgman et al., used an obsolete 0.15 tesla magnet MRI device and reported that CT was more accurate than this MRI device. The other two studies used more modern MRI machines and reported higher accuracy rates for MRI than for CT for rectal T staging, but the results did not reach statistical significance (Figure 6). This may be due to lack of power, as the accuracy analysis only included 40 patients, and the understaging and overstaging data come from one small study each.

One study by Barbaro et al.[92] compared CT, MRI, and ERUS for rectal T staging. The data reported by this study are shown in Appendix C. The authors concluded that for rectal T staging, ERUS was most accurate, MRI was slightly less accurate than ERUS, and CT was less accurate than either MRI or ERUS.

Table 13. Summary results for primary preoperative rectal T staging

Test Characteristics	MRI vs. ERUS	ERUS vs. CT	MRI vs. CT
Sensitivity (95% CI) of T1/T2 vs. T3/T4	MRI: 88.9% (79.0% to 94.4%) ERUS: 88.0% (80.0% to 93.1%)	Not calculated	Not calculated
Specificity (95% CI) of T1/T2 vs. T3/T4	MRI: 85.3% (70.6% to 93.4%) ERUS: 85.6% (65.8% to 94.9%)	Not calculated	Not calculated
Accuracy: OR of getting an incorrect result (95% CI)[a]	1.24 (0.835 to 1.84)	0.359 (0.238 to 0.541)	0.317 (0.056 to 1.784)[b]
Understaging OR (95% CI)[a]	1.571 (0.605 to 4.083)	0.626 (0.438 to 0.894)	0.317 (0.027 to 3.646) (based on Guinet et al.[113], n=19)
Overstaging OR (95% CI)[a]	1.05 (0.518 to 2.16)	0.472 (0.28 to 0.798)	0.317 (0.028 to 3.653) (based on Matsuoka et al. 2003[112], n=21)
Favors	No statistical difference	ERUS	No statistical difference

CI=Confidence interval; CT=computed tomography; ERUS=endorectal ultrasound; MRI=magnetic resonance imaging.

[a] OR < 1 indicates a lower risk of error in the first imaging modality listed in the column header; OR > 1 indicates a higher risk of error in the first imaging modality listed in the column header.

[b] Study with 0.15T magnet excluded from analyses.

Figure 3. MRI versus ERUS accuracy for rectal T staging

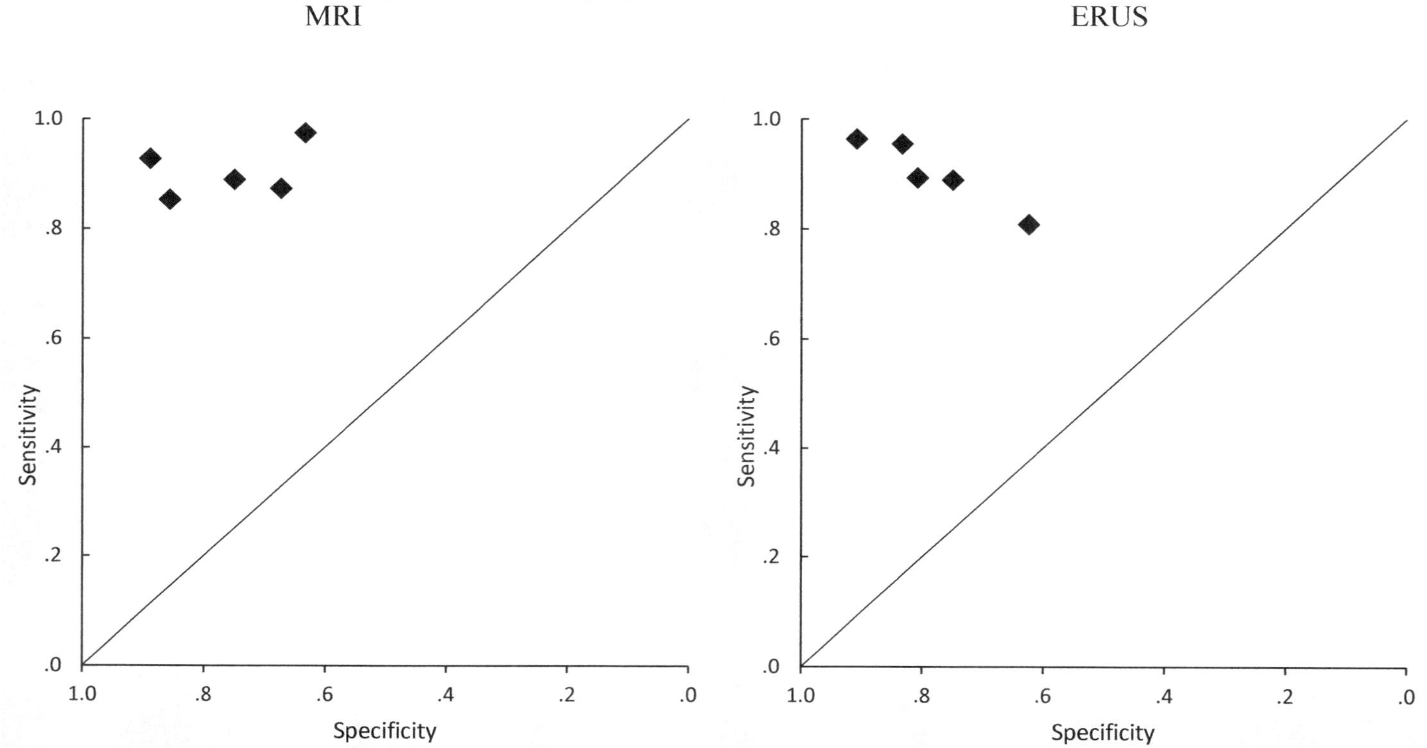

Graphical representation in ROC space of reported data for MRI (left side) vs. ERUS (right side) for rectal T staging. The data points for each study are shown as black diamonds. The diagonal line represents chance.

Figure 4. CT versus ERUS: risk of rectal T overstaging

Study name	Odds ratio	Lower limit	Upper limit
Ju	0.157	0.066	0.375
Kim	0.963	0.499	1.856
Osti	0.859	0.400	1.846
Goldman	0.420	0.161	1.095
Rotte	0.306	0.053	1.749
Beynon	0.651	0.175	2.419
Kramann	0.284	0.081	0.998
Romano	0.477	0.079	2.866
	0.472	0.280	0.798

Figure 5. CT versus ERUS: risk of rectal T understaging

Study name	Odds ratio	Lower limit	Upper limit
Ju	0.567	0.264	1.215
Kim	0.842	0.427	1.660
Osti	0.542	0.216	1.362
Goldman	0.284	0.081	0.998
Pappalar	0.462	0.074	2.865
Rotte	1.568	0.410	5.999
Beynon	0.371	0.107	1.294
Kramann	0.322	0.028	3.669
Romano	1.000	0.234	4.265
	0.626	0.438	0.894

Figure 6. MRI versus CT rectal T accuracy

Study name	Odds ratio	Lower limit	Upper limit	Z-Value	p-Value
Matsuoka	0.318	0.028	3.653	-0.920	0.358
Guinet	0.316	0.027	3.646	-0.923	0.356
	0.317	0.056	1.784	-1.303	0.193

Odds ratio and 95% CI: 0.1 0.2 0.5 1 2 5 10 — Favors MRI | Favors CT

Two studies (Blomqvist et al.[115] and Fleshman et al.[116]) also reported on the accuracy of staging performed before neoadjuvant therapy, using surgery after the treatment as the reference standard. The lag time and treatment given may confound the results of these studies—namely, the pretreatment stage may have been correctly identified by the imaging modality, but by the time surgery/histopathology had been performed, the patient's stage may have changed. The Blomqvist study compared MRI with CT in a retrospective analysis of patients with locally advanced cancer who underwent neoadjuvant chemotherapy before surgery. The data reported by the study are shown in Appendix C. The accuracy of both CT and MRI was reported to be quite poor (44.4% and 46.2%, respectively) but should be interpreted carefully because of the potentially confounding factors. The Fleshman study compared CT with ERUS in a prospective study of patients with advanced rectal tumors who underwent neoadjuvant radiation therapy before surgery. Similar to the other study, Fleshman reported that both modalities had very poor accuracy for pretreatment T staging (53% for CT and 32% for ERUS), but had excellent accuracy for N staging (both modalities had 100% negative predictive value for affected lymph nodes). Again, the results should be interpreted carefully because of the potentially confounding factors.

Preoperative Rectal Nodal Staging

We identified 19 studies that reported data on rectal N staging (summarized in Table 14). One study compared MRI with PET/CT, five compared MRI with ERUS, nine compared CT with ERUS, and four compared MRI with CT.

Kim et al. compared MRI with PET/CT for rectal N staging. The data reported by Kim et al. are shown in Appendix C. MRI had superior sensitivity over PET/CT for detecting affected lymph nodes (94% vs. 61%, respectively), but PET/CT had a higher specificity (83% vs. 67%, respectively). The authors concluded that MRI is preferable for rectal N node staging because missing affected lymph nodes is a more clinically serious error than false-positive findings.

Table 14. Preoperative rectal nodal staging

Study	Compares	Number of Patients	Design	Risk of Bias
Kim et al. 2011[88]	MRI to PET/CT	30	Retrospective cohort	Moderate
Yimei et al. 2012[93]	MRI to ERUS	129	Retrospective controlled trial	Moderate
Halefoglu et al. 2008[94]	MRI to ERUS	34	Cohort	Low
Bianchi et al. 2005[95]	MRI to ERUS	49	Cohort	Moderate
Starck et al. 1995[96]	MRI to ERUS	35	Prospective cohort	Moderate
Thaler et al. 1994[97]	MRI to ERUS	34	Prospective cohort	Low
Ju et al. 2009[99]	CT to ERUS	78	Cohort	Moderate
Kim et al. 1999[100]	CT to ERUS	89	Cohort	Moderate
Osti et al. 1997[101]	CT to ERUS	63	Cohort	Moderate
Ramana et al. 1997[102]	CT to ERUS	10	Prospective cohort	Moderate
Goldman et al. 1991[103]	CT to ERUS	29	Prospective cohort	Moderate
Pappalardo et al. 1990[104]	CT to ERUS	14	Prospective cohort	Moderate
Rotte et al. 1989[105]	CT to ERUS	25	Cohort	Moderate
Rifkin and Wechsler 1986[109]	CT to ERUS	79	Prospective cohort	Moderate
Rifkin, McGlynn, and Marks 1986[110]	CT to ERUS	54	Prospective cohort	Moderate
Arii et al. 2004[117]	MRI to CT	53	Prospective cohort	Moderate
Matsuoka et al. 2003[112]	MRI to CT	21	Prospective cohort	Moderate

Table 14. Preoperative rectal nodal staging, (continued)

Study	Compares	Number of Patients	Design	Risk of Bias
Guinet et al. 1990[113]	MRI to CT	19	Cohort	Moderate
Hodgman et al. 1986[114]	MRI to CT	30	Cohort	Moderate

CT=Computed tomography; ERUS=endorectal ultrasound; MRI=magnetic resonance imaging.

The data reported by the five studies that compared MRI with ERUS for rectal N staging are shown in Appendix C. We pooled the data in a binomial-bivariate regression model; full details of the results and HSROC curves are shown in Appendix D. We also pooled the accuracy, over-, and understaged data in random-effects models. The full details of these results are shown in Appendix D. The results of the analyses are summarized below, in Table 15. The bivariate model suggests that ERUS had a slightly higher sensitivity and specificity than MRI, but the confidence intervals overlap, indicating the difference is probably not significant. The accuracy, overstaging and understaging comparisons of ERUS and MRI did not find statistically significant differences. Therefore, we conclude that for preoperative rectal N staging, MRI and ERUS are similar in accuracy. The level of study limitations was medium; the data were consistent and direct but not precise (wide confidence intervals), so the strength of evidence supporting this conclusion is low.

The data reported by the nine studies that compared CT with ERUS are shown in Appendix C. We pooled the data in a binomial-bivariate regression model; full details of the results and HSROC curves are shown in Appendix D. We also pooled the accuracy, over-, and understaging data in random-effects models. The full details of these results are shown in in Appendix D. The results are summarized in Table 15, below. The bivariate model indicates no significant differences in sensitivity or specificity. The results of the accuracy, over-, and understaging analyses also indicated no significant difference. The level of study limitations was medium; the data were consistent and direct but not precise (wide confidence intervals), so the strength of evidence supporting this conclusion is low.

The data reported by the four studies that compared MRI with CT are shown in Appendix C. Because only three of the four reported sensitivity and specificity, we did not compute a bivariate model. However, we pooled the data for accuracy, over-, and understaging in a random-effects model. The full results are shown in Appendix D and summarized below in Table 15. The accuracy analysis indicated no significant difference between the two modalities; however, MRI is less likely than CT to overstage (OR = 0.498, 95% CI, 0.308 to 0.806). CT appears to be less likely to understage than is MRI, but the result did not remain statistically significant in sensitivity analyses when we varied the correlation for tests performed in the same subjects. Table 16 provides a list of factors we considered that may have impacted the results, but we did not have sufficient data to explore this further.

Table 16. Summary results for rectal N staging

Test Characteristics	MRI vs. ERUS	CT vs. ERUS	MRI vs. CT
Sensitivity (95% CI)	MRI: 49.5% (36.0% to 63.1%) ERUS: 53.0% (39.7% to 65.5%)	CT: 39.6% (28.1% to 52.4%) ERUS: 49.1% (34.9% to 63.5%)	Not calculated
Specificity (95% CI)	MRI: 69.7% (51.9% to 83.0%) ERUS: 73.7% (43.6% to 91.0%)	CT: 93.2% (58.8% to 99.2%) ERUS: 71.7% (56.2% to 83.4%)	Not calculated
Accuracy: OR of getting an incorrect result (95% CI)[a]	0.882 (0.542 to 1.408)	1.13 (0.85 to 1.503)	1.316 (0.709 to 2.443)
Understaging OR (95% CI)[a]	0.972 (0.563 to 1.679)	1.453 (0.854 to 2.473)	1.743 (1.028 to 2.957) (not robust in sensitivity analysis)
Overstaging OR (95% CI)[a]	0.752 (0.457 to 1.237)	1.015 (0.571 to 1.801)	0.498 (0.308 to 0.806)
Favors	Not statistically different	Not statistically different	CT favored for avoiding understaging, and MRI favored for avoiding overstaging

CI=Confidence interval; CT=computed tomography; ERUS=endorectal ultrasound; MRI=magnetic resonance imaging.

[a]OR < 1 indicates a lower risk of error in the first imaging modality listed in the column header; OR > 1 indicates a higher risk of error in the first imaging modality listed in the column header.

Table 17. Rectal N staging: differences between studies in various factors

Factor	MRI vs. ERUS	CT vs. ERUS	MRI vs. CT
Date of publication	40% before 2000 60% after 2005	88% before 2000 11% after 2005	33% before 2000 0 after 2005
Patient age	Mean: 58.7 to 68 years	67% did not report	Means 62 to 66 years
Percentage of male patients	44.1% to 68%	54% to 70%	58.8% to 74%
CT details	Not applicable	22% rectal air 11% rectal contrast 56% oral contrast 33% IV contrast 11% bowel prep	25% rectal air 50% rectal contrast 50% oral contrast 100% IV contrast 25% bowel prep
MRI details	20% rectal air 0% IV contrast 20% bowel prep 20% 3T magnet 50% 1.0 and 1.5T magnets 20% 0.3T magnet 100% T2 weighting 60% T1 weighting	Not applicable	50% rectal air 25% IV contrast 25% bowel prep 50% 1.5T magnet 25% 0.5T magnet 25% 0.15T magnet 100% T2 weighting 100% T1 weighting

CT=Computed tomography; IV=intravenous; MRI=magnetic resonance imaging; T=tesla

Preoperative Recurrent Rectal Staging

One study reported on staging recurrent rectal cancer (Milsom et al.[118]). The study included a prospective comparison of CT with ERUS for staging of biopsy-proven, recurrent rectal cancer in 14 patients. The data are presented in Appendix C. The authors reported that ERUS was better than CT for predicting the extent of local organ invasion (i.e., bladder, rectum, prostate). However, one small (n=14) study is insufficient to support an evidence-based conclusion.

Preoperative Rectal Circumferential Margin Status

Only one study reported information about assessing circumferential margin (CRM) status. The study directly compared MRI with CT for this purpose (Taylor et al.[119]). The study was retrospective in design and examined the records of 42 patients, who were examined by T1- and T2-weighted 1.5T MRI with a phased-array coil and CT using intravenous contrast; no intravenous contrast agent was used for the MRI examinations. See Table C-42 in Appendix C for the reported data. CT was reported to be more accurate than MRI in assessing CRM status (64.3% vs. 54.8%, respectively); the authors concluded that both modalities tended to overstage CRM status but rarely understage it. The study was rated as being at moderate risk of bias, but a single study is insufficient to support an evidence-based conclusion.

Preoperative Colon Staging

We did not identify any studies of staging that enrolled patients who had only colon cancer (not mixed with rectal cancer cases) that met the inclusion criteria.

Preoperative Colorectal Tumor Staging

We identified only one study that reported on preoperative colorectal T staging (Uchiyama et al.[89]). The study was a prospective comparison of CT versus PET/CT on a mixed group of patients with rectal and colon cancer. See Appendix C for the data reported by this study. The authors reported that PET/CT was to be preferred for T staging because it had a higher accuracy (95.0% vs. 78.8%, respectively). Rates of over- and understaging were not reported, nor was the sensitivity or specificity of the modalities for distinguishing between T1/T2 stages and T3/T4 stages. A single study is insufficient to support an evidence-based conclusion.

Preoperative Colorectal Nodal Staging

We identified only one study that reported on preoperative colorectal N staging (Uchiyama et al.[89]). The study was a prospective comparison of CT versus PET/CT in a mixed group of patients with rectal and colon cancer. See Appendix C for the data reported by this study. The authors reported that CT was preferable over PET/CT for N staging because it had a much higher sensitivity for detecting patients with affected lymph nodes (68.6% vs. 34.3%, respectively), although PET/CT was better than CT at identifying patients without affected lymph nodes (100% and 72.5% specificity, respectively). Although the study was rated as moderate risk of bias, a single study is insufficient to support an evidence-based conclusion.

Preoperative Colorectal Metastasis Staging

We identified nine studies of preoperative colorectal M staging (summarized in Table 17). Four compared PET/CT with CT, and five compared MRI with CT.

Unlike the other studies of PET/CT versus CT, Uchiyama et al. enrolled patients for T, N, and M staging; the other studies enrolled patients to specifically look for suspected liver metastases; therefore, we decided to not include Uchiyama in the meta-analysis. Lubezky et al. reported data on a per-patient basis, and the other two remaining studies reported data on a per-lesion basis. We therefore decided to pool only the data from Orlacchio et al. and Ramos et al. in a random-effects meta-analysis of sensitivity for detecting colorectal liver metastases (per lesion basis). See Appendix C for the data reported by all four studies.

We were able to calculate the lesion detection rate on a per-lesion basis for all five studies of MRI versus CT; therefore, we pooled data from all five in a random-effects meta-analysis. See Appendix C for the data reported by these studies.

Table 17. Preoperative colorectal M staging

Study	Compares	Number of Patients	Design	Risk of Bias
Uchiyama et al. 2012[89]	PET/CT to CT	77 colorectal	Prospective cohort	Moderate
Ramos et al. 2011[19]	PET/CT to CT	70 colorectal	Prospective cohort	Moderate
Orlacchio et al. 2009[90]	PET/CT to CT	467 colorectal	Cohort	Moderate
Lubezky et al. 2007[91]	PET/CT to CT	27 colorectal	Cohort	Moderate
Bartolozzi et al. 2004[120]	MRI to CT	44 colorectal	Prospective cohort	Low
Bhattacharjya et al. 2004[121]	MRI to CT	100 colorectal	Prospective cohort	Moderate
Bohm et al. 2004[122]	MRI to CT	24 colorectal	Prospective cohort	Moderate
Lencioni et al. 1998[123]	MRI to CT	14 colorectal	Prospective cohort	Low
Strotzer et al. 1997[124]	MRI to CT	35 colorectal	Prospective cohort	Low

CT=computed tomography; MRI=magnetic resonance imaging; PET/CT=positron emission tomography/computed tomography.

The results of the two meta-analyses are summarized in Table 18. MRI was superior to CT, and the difference was statistically significant. CT was superior to PET/CT, and the confidence intervals around the summary effect measure did not overlap, suggesting the difference is statistically significant. The level of study limitations for the CT-versus-MRI data set was low. The data were consistent and direct but not precise. Thus, we graded the overall strength of evidence for MRI versus CT as moderate. For PET/CT versus CT, the level of study limitations was medium; but the results were neither consistent nor precise, so we graded the strength of evidence supporting that conclusion as insufficient.

Table 18. Pooled random-effects analyses for preoperative colorectal M staging (per lesion basis)

Measure	CT vs. MRI	PET/CT vs. CT
Sensitivity	Not calculated	CT: 83.6% (95% CI, 78.1% to 88.2%) PET/CT: 60.4% (95% CI, 53.7% to 66.9%)
Summary OR for lesion detection rate[a]	1.334 (95% CI 1.012 to 1.761)	Not calculated
I^2	36%	CT: 0.0% PET/CT: 95.1%
Favors	MRI	Insufficient evidence

CI=Confidence interval; CT=computed tomography; MRI=magnetic resonance imaging; PET/CT=positron emission tomography/computed tomography.

OR > 1 indicates greater likelihood of detecting metastatic lesions by the first imaging modality in the column header.

Comparative and Additive Impact of Imaging Modalities on Stage Reclassification and Management

Key Question 1b. What is the impact of alternative imaging techniques on intermediate outcomes, including stage reclassification and changes in therapeutic management?

Key Points

- MRI and ERUS were assessed for primary rectal cancer treatment decisionmaking but pooled results were not statistically significant.
- Addition of ERUS to CT during primary rectal cancer treatment resulted in changes in management, but appropriateness was not assessed. Strength of evidence was graded as insufficient.
- Addition of PET/CT to CT for preoperative rectal cancer staging resulted in changes in management, but in the one study measuring appropriateness, changes were appropriate in only half of the instances. Strength of evidence was graded as insufficient.

Detailed Synthesis

Magnetic Resonance Imaging Versus Endorectal Ultrasound

Two studies that met the inclusion criteria reported on patient management based on MRI or ERUS for preoperative rectal staging (Yimea et al.[93] and Brown et al.[125]). Both studies used a similar design: for each patient, the investigators devised a theoretical treatment strategy based solely on MRI information, they devised another theoretical treatment strategy based solely on ERUS information, and then they used a third strategy based on clinical information, MRI, and ERUS data to actually treat the patient. The histopathology after surgery was used to define the "correct" treatment strategy that should have been used. See Appendix C for the results reported by the studies. We pooled the results from both studies in a random-effects meta-analysis. We analyzed the outcomes "correct treatment," "undertreatment," and "overtreatment." All three analyses favored MRI as the more accurate modality for treatment planning, but none reached statistical significance. See Appendix D for details of the meta-analyses.

Endorectal Ultrasound Added to Computed Tomography Staging

Two studies that met the inclusion criteria reported the impact of adding ERUS information to CT results for preoperative staging of rectal cancer (Wickramasinghe and Samarasekera[126] and Harewood et al.[127]). One study reported that 25 percent of patients had a change in management after adding the ERUS information, but whether the change was appropriate was not measured or reported. The other study reported that 31 percent of patients had a change in management after adding the ERUS information, primarily changes from surgery to neoadjuvant therapy. Whether the changes were appropriate was not measured or reported. For more information, see Appendix C. Because of the lack of measuring whether the changes were appropriate, we graded this evidence base as insufficient to support an evidence-based conclusion.

Positron Emission Tomography/Computed Tomography Added to Conventional Staging

Two studies that met the inclusion criteria reported the impact of adding PET/CT results to CT results for preoperative staging of colorectal cancer (Engledow et al.[128] and Ramos et al.[19]). Engledow et al. reported that adding PET/CT results changed management for 34 percent of the patients, but whether the change was appropriate was not measured or reported. Ramos et al. reported that adding PET/CT to CT results changed management for 17.5 percent of patients, but after treatment, surgery, and followup, results indicated that only half of the changed treatment plans were the appropriate choice. For more information, see Appendix C.

One study (Eglinton et al.[129]) examined 19 patients with rectal cancer for preoperative staging with PET/CT, MRI, CT, and clinical information and developed a treatment plan in-house. The information from the MRI, CT, and clinical information, but not the PET/CT information, was sent to a different institution, where a treatment plan was developed. The two treatment plans were compared. Minor changes were made to treatment plans for five patients, most of whom had stage IV cancer. The appropriateness of the changes was not measured or reported. For more information, see Appendix C. Because only one study measured the appropriateness of the treatment plan changes, we graded the evidence base as insufficient to support an evidence-based conclusion.

Comparative and Additive Impact of Imaging Modalities on Clinical Outcomes

Key Question 1c. What is the impact of alternative imaging techniques on clinical outcomes?

We did not identify any studies that addressed the question of the impact of alternative imaging techniques on clinical outcomes.

Adverse Effects Associated With Imaging Techniques

Key Question 1d. What are the adverse effects or harms associated with using imaging techniques, including harms of test-directed management?

Key Points

- Serious adverse effects are rare with ERUS, but patients do report varying degrees of discomfort during the procedure, and some procedures cannot be completed due to presence of strictures, stenosis or angulation of the rectum.
- Rare but potential harms of MRI are associated with use of gadolinium-based contrast agents.
- Harms of CT include radiation exposure and adverse events from intravenous contrast agents.
- Harms from PET/CT include radiation exposure from the CT component and from the tracer used for PET.

Detailed Synthesis

To address the question of harm associated with using imaging techniques, we abstracted data about harms reported by the included studies (see Appendix C). We supplemented this information with information from narrative reviews and other sources (e.g., U.S. Food and Drug Administration [FDA] alerts). Additionally, we systematically searched for information on harms related to the imaging modalities of interest (regardless of condition or disease state). Our search strategy is shown in Appendix A. Our searches identified 1,961 abstracts; after review of these abstracts, we selected 66 articles to review in full text. Our inclusion criteria for the supplemental harms searches were that the articles must have been published in English and specifically focused on adverse events from CT, MRI, PET/CT, or ERUS in any patient population. Clinical studies must have been published in 2008 or later, and narrative reviews must have been published in 2012 or later. After full-text review, we included 32 studies reporting on general harms from CT[130-144], ERUS[145-149], MRI[140,150-160], and PET/CT.[140,161]

We did not grade the strength of evidence for harms because we combined information drawn from a wide range of sources.

Endorectal Ultrasound

Ultrasound is generally considered to be extremely safe. Ultrasound examinations that use microbubble contrast agents have the potential for patients to react to the agents, but most reactions appear to be transient and mild, consisting of alteration of taste, facial flushing, and pain at the injection site; however, contrast agents are rarely if ever used for ERUS.[162] As long as routine practices are followed, ultrasound imaging can generally be considered a safe exam for most patients.

For colorectal imaging, an additional consideration is the fact that an endorectal probe is inserted into the rectum. Possible complications include perforation, bleeding, and pain. The majority of included studies of ERUS did not report any complications; whether this means that none occurred is unclear. Six studies reported adverse events. One study (Rifkin et al.[110]) reported that all 51 patients experienced mild discomfort during the procedure. One study (Milsom et al.[118]) measured the level of discomfort experienced using a visual analog scale and reported the mean discomfort level as a 3 (with a 10 representing maximal pain). Three studies (Pomerri et al.[163], Huh et al.[164], and Brown et al.[125]) reported that some (11% to 38%) of the patients experienced severe pain during the procedure. Two studies (Rifkin and Wechsler[109] and Rifkin et al.[110]) reported some (4% to 10%) patients had minor rectal bleeding after the procedure. ERUS cannot be performed in some patients because of tight stenosis or the lesion being too far from the anal verge. Four of the studies reported instances of incomplete procedures due to strictures, stenosis or angulations.[96,97,105,165] (See Appendix C.)

The supplemental harms searches identified a narrative review of complications of endoscopic ultrasound, including ERUS.[17] The authors commented on the rarity of ERUS-related perforation, and noted that only one case had been reported in a prospective registry of the German Society of Ultrasound in Medicine.[17] While the multicenter registry includes nearly 12,000 endoscopic ultrasound examinations, the number of ERUS procedures was not reported in the review.

Computed Tomography

None of the included studies reported any adverse events related to CT.

CT scans expose the body to x-rays. A typical abdominal CT scan exposes the body to approximately 10 mSv of radiation.[166] Cadwallader et al.[136] reported results from 198 scans of at-risk patients to determine the risk of fatal cancer induction. Forty-one (20.7%) scans did not alter management of the patient and were thus deemed as unnecessarily exposing patients to CT radiation. According to the National Cancer Institute, the extra risk of one person for developing a fatal cancer from the radiation from a single CT procedure is about 1 in 2,000.[167]

The supplemental harms searches identified 15 studies of more than 190,000 patients reported on CT-related adverse events (all related to the administration of contrast agents).[130-144] Most studies administered nonionic contrast agents, whereas two studies administered iothalamate meglumine, an ionic contrast agent.[141,143] Nonionic contrast agents, introduced in the 1970s, have a lower osmolarity than blood and are therefore less likely to cause adverse reactions.[144] Nonionic contrast agents evaluated included iopromide,[130,133,140,141,144] iomeprol,[130,131,144] iohexol,[130,131,138] iopamidol,[131,132,137,139,144] iodixanol,[130,139] and ioversol.[131,135,141,144]

Three of the 15 studies reported only mild-to-moderate harms,[130,139,143] but eight of the 15 studies reported serious/severe adverse events.[131,134,135,137,140-142,144] Two studies reported 25 deaths within 30[142] to 45 days[134] after CT. Weisbord[142] enrolled 421 patients thought to be at increased risk of developing contrast-induced acute kidney injury and reported 10 (2.4% of patients) deaths within 30 days after imaging.

Kobayashi et al.[131] reported 23 (0.06%) severe reactions to contrast agents, including shock, hypotension, desaturation, and airway obstruction in a retrospective cohort study of 36,472 patients. Patients received various nonionic low-osmolar contrast agents; approximately half of the study population was diabetic (19.5%) or hypertensive (28.6%). Vogl et al.[135] reported anaphylactoid adverse reactions requiring hospitalization in 4 (0.03%) patients receiving ioversol. Jung et al.[144] focused on cutaneous adverse reactions in 47,388 patients receiving various nonionic monomers such as iomeprol. Severe reactions such as severe generalized urticaria and facial edema occurred in 16 patients. The three remaining studies reported shortness of breath (5 patients)[140] and one case each of atrial fibrillation (patient on peritoneal dialysis),[137] cyanosis,[141] and severe laryngeal edema.[141] See Appendix C for details on CT-related adverse events.

Magnetic Resonance Imaging

A patient undergoing an MRI exam faces many well-known safety hazards, including patient heating, pacemaker malfunction, dislodgment of metallic implants, peripheral nerve stimulation, acoustic noise, and radiofrequency-induced burns.[168-173] MRI facilities take precautions to routinely screen patients for possible contraindications. Patients are routinely asked to wear earplugs and are given an emergency call button. No adverse effects have been conclusively identified in association with the magnetic fields to which patients are exposed during routine MRI scanning.[174-177] Therefore, if routine precautions are followed, MRI can be considered a safe exam for most patients. A search for reports of patient discomfort did not find any reports of severe discomfort. In fact, to decrease patient motion, it is important that the patient be as comfortable as possible.[45]

Only two of the included studies reported adverse events due to MRI, both of which were of patients refusing the procedure due to severe claustrophobia (Pomerri et al.[163] and Bhattacharjya et al.[121]).

The supplemental harms searches identified 12 studies of more than 157,000 patients reporting on MRI-related harms.[140,150-160] Adverse events from contrast-enhanced MRIs were the focus of 11 (92%) of the 12 studies.[140,150,151,153-160] See Appendix C for a list and description of the currently marketed contrast agents for MRI. Contrast-enhanced MRIs, widely used for more than 20 years, provide increased sensitivity and specificity of lesion detection.[178] Although relatively safe in most patients, contrast agents may be quite harmful to others.

The American College of Radiology's (ACR) "ACR Manual on Contrast Media" (2013) indicates that patients with a history of earlier allergy-like reaction to contrast media, history of asthma, renal insufficiency, significant cardiac disease, and elevated anxiety are at an increased risk for adverse intravenous contrast material reactions.[179] Some reactions may be life threatening or potentially fatal. In 2006, some gadolinium-based contrast agents (GBCAs) were linked with nephrogenic systemic fibrosis (NSF), a scleroderma-like, fibrosing condition, that could be potentially fatal in patients with renal failure.[180] NSF is a progressive, disabling, and potentially fatal disorder that leads to deposition of excessive connective tissue in the skin and internal organs. The condition was previously unknown; the typical patient is a middle-aged individual with severe renal disease who first exhibits skin changes 2–4 weeks after undergoing an MRI examination that used gadolinium-based contrast agents.[181]

The ACR manual[179] estimates that "patients with end-stage chronic kidney disease (CKD) (CKD5, eGFR <15 ml/min/1.73 m^2) and severe CKD (CKD4, eGFR 15 to 29 ml/min/1.73 m^2) have a 1 percent to 7 percent chance of developing NSF after one or more exposures to at least some GBCAs." In 2010, FDA issued a warning about using GBCAs in patients with kidney dysfunction. Agents such as Magnevist, Omiscan, and OptiMark, FDA states, place certain patients with kidney dysfunction at higher risk for NSF than other GBCAs.[182] FDA had previously issued a Public Health Advisory (2006) about the possible link between exposure to GBCAs for magnetic resonance angiography and NSF in patients with kidney failure.[183] The FDA later (2007) required a box warning on product labeling of all GBCAs used in MRIs regarding the risk of NSF in patients with severe kidney insufficiency, patients just before or just after liver transplantation, or individuals with chronic liver disease.[184]

The largest study of MRI adverse events that we identified (n=84,621) included 19,354 (22.9%) patients with renal and liver dysfunctions, history of allergies, hypertension, chronic heart disease, and central nervous system disorders. All patients in this study received injections of gadolinium-based contrast agents.[153] Four hundred twenty-one adverse events (65 different types) occurred in 285 out of the 84,621 patients (0.34%). Eight serious (3 life-threatening) adverse events (less than 0.01%) were reported.

See Appendix C for details on MRI-related adverse events.

Positron Emission Tomography/Computed Tomography

Using a typical dose of tracer (400 MBq) for a whole-body scan, the effective radiation dose delivered during a typical PET study is 7.6 mSv. The use of a combined CT/PET scanner also exposes the patient to x-rays. A typical abdominal CT scan exposes the body to approximately 10 mSv, for a total of around 18 mSv for a single PET/CT study.[166] Studies of atomic-bomb survivors and radiation workers have found a significant increase in the risk of cancer after exposure to as little as 20 mSv.[166] Therefore, radiation dose from PET/CT scans may be a health concern. After the exam, the short half-life of ^{18}F means that additional precautions, such as avoiding public transportation, are not necessary.[185]

None of the included studies reported any adverse events related to PET/CT.

The supplemental harms searches identified two studies of 3,360 patients that reported on PET/CT-related harms.[140,161] Codreanu et al.[161] reported mild harms (recurring body rash and itching from ^{18}F-fluorodeoxyglucose) in one male patient with pyriform sinus cancer and history of allergies. A retrospective review of 3,359 PET/CT scans (106,800 scans overall)[140] reported four severe adverse events, including chest pain (2 patients) and shortness of breath (2 patients). See Appendix C for PET/CT-related harms.

Factors Affecting Accuracy

Key Question 1e. How is the comparative effectiveness of imaging techniques modified by the following factors: patient-level characteristics (e.g., age, sex, body mass index); disease characteristics (e.g., tumor grade); and imaging technique or protocol characteristics (e.g., use of different tracers or contrast agents, radiation dose of the imaging modality, slice thickness, timing of contrast)?

Key Points

- Only single studies addressed each of several factors affecting accuracy of ERUS for colorectal staging; the evidence was graded as insufficient.
- Only single studies addressed each of several factors affecting accuracy of CT for colorectal cancer staging; the evidence was graded as insufficient.

Detailed Synthesis

Endorectal Ultrasound

Five studies reported factors affecting the accuracy of ERUS for colorectal staging (see Appendix C for details). Kim et al.[186] reported that ERUS was more accurate for rectal T and N staging if the rectum was filled with water. Mo et al.[165] reported that a miniprobe was slightly less accurate than a conventional probe for colorectal T staging, but the conventional probe was much more accurate than a miniprobe for colorectal N staging. Hunerbein et al.[187] reported that three-dimensional (3D) ERUS was slightly more accurate than two-dimensional (2D) ERUS for rectal T staging. Huh et al.[164] reported that ERUS was much more accurate for rectal T staging when the tumor was located closer to the anal verge. Rafaelsen et al.[188] reported that experienced readers were more accurate than inexperienced readers for rectal T and N staging. Because only one study reported on each factor, we graded the evidence base as insufficient to support an evidence-based conclusion.

Computed Tomography

Three studies reported factors affecting the accuracy of CT for colorectal staging (see Appendix C for more details). Skriver et al.[189] reported that using intravenous contrast material did not improve CT's accuracy for rectal T and N staging. Lupo et al.[190] reported that filling the rectum with water improved CT's accuracy for rectal T staging. Wicherts et al.[191] reported that arterial and equilibrium-phase CT did not add any additional information to hepatic venous-phase CT for colorectal liver M staging. Because only one study reported on each factor, we graded the evidence base as insufficient to support an evidence-based conclusion.

Magnetic Resonance Imaging

Nine studies reported factors affecting the accuracy of MRI for colorectal staging (see Appendix C for more details). Rafaelsen et al.[188] reported that experienced readers were more accurate than inexperienced readers for rectal T and N staging. Koh et al.[192] reported that diffusion-weighted MRI was slightly more accurate than contrast-enhanced T1-/T2-weighted MRI for colorectal M staging. Jao et al. (2010)[193] and Vliegen et al. (2005)[194] compared gadolinium-enhanced T1-weighted MRI to T2-weighted MRI. Jao reported that the addition of contrast did not improve rectal T and N staging. Vliegen reported that contrast did not improve T staging and did not report data on N staging. Okizuka et al. (1996)[195] reported that gadopentetate dimeglumine enhanced fat-suppressed MRI imaging was not better than conventional T1-and T2-weighted MRI for rectal T and N staging.

One study (Kim et al.[196]) reported that 2D and 3D T2-weighted imaging were equally accurate for rectal N and T staging, but Futterer et al.[197] reported that 3D imaging was less accurate than 2D imaging for rectal T staging, and more motion artifacts appeared. Kim et al.[196] reported that filling the rectum with water improved the accuracy of rectal T staging but did not affect the accuracy of rectal N staging.

In regard to colorectal M staging, Koh et al.[192] reported that diffusion-weighted MRI was slightly more accurate than contrast-enhanced T1-/T2-weighted MRI for colorectal M staging, but that the combination was superior.

For cases in which only one study reported on each factor, we graded the evidence base as insufficient to support an evidence-based conclusion.

Two studies reported on 2D versus 3D imaging; the level of study limitations was judged to be medium, but because the evidence was inconsistent and a quantitative analysis could not be performed, we graded the evidence base as insufficient to support an evidence-based conclusion.

Three studies reported that contrast-enhancement did not improve the accuracy of MRI for rectal T and N staging. The level of study limitations of this evidence base was rated as low, and the evidence was qualitatively consistent and direct; however, a quantitative analysis could not be performed. We did not grade the strength of evidence for this outcome.

Positron Emission Tomography/Computed Tomography

No studies reported factors that affected the accuracy of PET/CT.

Conclusions for Key Question 1

We compiled data from recent, high-quality systematic reviews to estimate the accuracy of each individual imaging modality in isolation (see Table 19 for a summary of these data). Because insufficient data existed on PET/CT from systematic reviews, we examined the studies of PET/CT included in this report to address the comparative questions to obtain an estimate of accuracy.

Table 19. Accuracy of imaging tests as reported by recent systematic reviews

Staging	ERUS	CT	MRI	PET/CT
Rectal T	For identifying T1: Sensitivity: 87.8% (85.3 to 90.0%) Specificity: 98.3% (97.8 to 98.7%) For identifying T2: Sensitivity: 80.5% (77.9 to 82.9%) Specificity: 95.6% (94.9 to 96.3%) For identifying T3: Sensitivity: 96.4% (95.4 to 97.2%) Specificity: 90.6% (89.5 to 91.7%) For identifying T4: Sensitivity: 95.4% (92.4 to 97.5%) Specificity: 98.3% (97.8 to 98.7%)	For distinguishing T1/T2 from T3/T4: Sensitivity: 86% (78 to 92%) Specificity: 78% (71 to 84%)	For distinguishing T1/T2 from T3/T4: Sensitivity: 87% (81 to 92%) Specificity: 75% (68 to 80%) For identifying affected CRM: Sensitivity: 77% (57 to 90%) Specificity: 94% (88 to 97%)	Not reported
Rectal N	For identifying affected nodes: Sensitivity: 73.2% (70.6 to 75.6%) Specificity: 75.8% (73.5 to 78.0%)	For identifying affected nodes: Sensitivity: 70% (59 to 80%) Specificity: 78% (66 to 86%)	For identifying affected nodes: Sensitivity: 77% (69 to 84%) Specificity: 71% (59 to 81%)	For identifying affected nodes: Sensitivity: 61% Specificity: 83%
Colorectal T	Mini-probe only: For identifying T1: Sensitivity: 91% (76 to 97%) Specificity: 98% (97 to 99%) For identifying T2: Sensitivity 78% (62 to 88%) Specificity: 94% (91 to 96%) For identifying T3+T4: Sensitivity: 97% (91 to 99%) Specificity: 90% (85 to 94%)	Not reported	Not reported	Accuracy: 95.0%
Colorectal N	Miniprobe only: For detecting affect nodes: Sensitivity 63% (47 to 77%) Specificity 82% (73 to 89%)	Not reported	Not reported	For identifying affected nodes: Sensitivity: 34.3% Specificity: 100%
Colorectal M	Not reported	For identifying liver metastases: Sensitivity 83.6%	For identifying liver metastases: Sensitivity: 88.2%	For identifying liver metastases: Sensitivity: 72% to 97.9%

CRM=Circumferential resection margin; CT=computed tomography; ERUS=endorectal ultrasound; M=metastases stage; MRI=magnetic resonance imaging; N=nodal stage; PET/CT=positron emission tomography/computed tomography; T=tumor stage; ( ) denotes the 95% confidence interval.

To determine the comparative effectiveness of the different modalities, we examined studies that directly compared modalities. For **rectal T staging**, ERUS is more accurate than CT (Strength of evidence is low.) ERUS and MRI appear to be similar in accuracy for rectal T staging as do MRI and CT (Strength of evidence is low.) The evidence was insufficient for drawing conclusions about the accuracy of PET/CT compared to either MRI or CT for rectal T staging.

For **rectal N staging**, ERUS, MRI, and CT all appear to be similar in accuracy, but they all have low sensitivity for detecting affected lymph nodes (upper bound of the confidence intervals for all 3 is less than 70%). MRI is less likely to overstage than is CT. (Strength of evidence is low.) The evidence was insufficient for drawing conclusions about the accuracy of PET/CT compared to either MRI or CT for rectal N staging.

For detecting **colorectal liver metastases**, MRI is superior to CT. (Strength of evidence is moderate.) The evidence was insufficient for drawing conclusions about the accuracy of PET/CT compared to either MRI or CT for colorectal M staging.

Three studies reported that contrast-enhancement did not improve the accuracy of MRI for rectal T and N staging. The level of study limitations of this evidence base was rated as low, and the evidence was qualitatively consistent and direct; however, a quantitative analysis could not be performed, and we did not assign an evidence grade.

The evidence base is characterized by a lack of studies reporting patient-oriented outcomes. Seven studies reported on the impact of imaging on patient management, but only three of these studies confirmed whether the change in management was appropriate. In general, the included studies reported only on diagnostic accuracy. They were all rated as either low or moderate risk of bias.

Too few studies exist for most of the evidence bases to allow a statistical analysis of the possibility of publication bias. However, because of reports that the ERUS literature, in particular, may be affected by publication bias, we have prepared funnel plots for the two larger ERUS evidence bases and have also run a meta-regression against publication date, all presented in Appendix D. While we recognize the limitations of funnel plots and of visual interpretation of them, the funnel plots do look fairly symmetrical. Also, there does not appear to be any pattern by date in the ERUS-versus-CT evidence base; there may be a tendency to report higher accuracy in older studies in the MRI-versus-ERUS evidence base, but the number of studies in that evidence base is too small to allow any conclusion to be reached.

Comparative Test Performance of Imaging Modalities for Restaging After Initial Treatment

Key Question 2. What is the comparative effectiveness of imaging techniques for restaging cancer in patients with primary and recurrent colorectal cancer after initial treatment?

> Key Question 2a. What is the test performance of the imaging techniques used (singly, in combination, or in a specific sequence) to restage colorectal cancer compared with a reference standard?

Key Points

As noted previously, interim restaging takes place after neoadjuvant chemotherapy and/or radiotherapy and in some cases, surgery. We attempted to address Key Question 2.a. using systematic reviews.

- We identified only one high-quality review of interim restaging that studied CT, MRI, and PET/CT for detecting colorectal liver metastases.
- MRI had a higher sensitivity for this purpose than the other modalities, but its sensitivity was still very low in this setting (69.9%, 95% CI: 65.6 to 73.9%).

Systematic Reviews

We identified only one recent (2009 or later) high-quality systematic review of interim restaging. Therefore, we searched for older high-quality systematic reviews of interim restaging but found none that that met the inclusion criteria.

The systematic review that met the inclusion criteria, van Kessel et al. 2012, included five studies of CT, two studies of MRI, and two studies of PET/CT. All studies evaluated patients who had undergone neoadjuvant chemotherapy followed by surgery or patient followup (approximately 8% of the patients did not undergo surgery). The sensitivities of detecting liver metastases in the interim restaging setting were calculated and pooled using random-effects or fixed-effects meta-analysis. See tables in Appendix C for details of this review's methodology. The findings are summarized below, in Table 20. The authors used visual analysis of funnel plots to check for publication bias and did not identify any evidence of publication bias in this literature base.

Table 20. Results from included systematic review of interim restaging

Study	Included Articles	Number of Patients	Primary Results	Author's Conclusion
Van Kessel et al. 2012[198]	5 CT 3 MRI 2 PET/CT	221 CT 54 MRI 137 PET/CT	Sensitivity for detecting colorectal liver metastases: CT 54.5% (95% CI, 46.7 to 62.1%) MRI 69.9% (95% CI, 65.6 to 73.9%) PET/CT 51.7% (95% CI, 37.8 to 65.4%)	MRI appears to be the most appropriate imaging modality for interim restaging of colorectal cancer liver metastases.

CT=computed tomography; MRI=magnetic resonance imaging; PET/CT=positron emission tomography/computed tomography

Detailed Synthesis

Interim Rectal Tumor Restaging

We identified four studies of interim rectal T staging (summarized in Table 21). One study compared CT with MRI, one compared CT with ERUS, and two compared MRI, ERUS, and CT.

Table 21. Interim rectal T restaging

Study	Compares	N Patients	Design	Risk of Bias
Blomqvist et al. 2002[115]	CT to MRI	15 with locally advanced rectal cancer	Retrospective cohort	Moderate
Huh et al. 2008[164]	CT to ERUS	83 with locally advanced rectal cancer within 7 cm of anal verge	Retrospective cohort	Low
Martellucci et al. 2012[199]	CT to ERUS to MRI	37 with locally advanced rectal cancer	Prospective cohort	Moderate
Pomerri et al. 2011[163]	CT to ERUS to MRI	90 with primary rectal cancer	Prospective cohort	Low

CT=Computed tomography; ERUS=endorectal ultrasound; MRI=magnetic resonance imaging.

The two studies of CT, ERUS, and MRI reported data differently enough that the only measure we were able to pool across the two studies was accuracy (i.e., we could not pool sensitivity, sensitivity, under- or over-staging). See Appendix C for the data reported by the studies. We pooled the reported accuracies using random-effects meta-analysis. See Appendix D for the results of the meta-analysis. Essentially, there was no difference in accuracy across the various modalities (MRI vs. CT, 0.943 (95% CI: 0.652 to 1.34), MRI vs. ERUS, 0.948 (95% CI: 0.471 to 1.907), CT vs. ERUS, 0.907 (95% CI: 0.41 to 2.011)).

Blomqvist et al. compared CT with MRI for restaging locally advanced cancer after neoadjuvant radiochemotherapy. See Appendix C for the data reported by the study. MRI had a better accuracy than CT (60.0% correctly staged vs. 41.7%, respectively), equivalent sensitivity for distinguishing between T1/T2 and T3/T4 stages (90%), but a much lower specificity (33.3% vs. 66.7%, respectively). The authors concluded that MRI was not significantly better than CT.

Huh et al. compared CT to ERUS for restaging locally advanced cancer after neoadjuvant radiochemotherapy. See Appendix C for the data reported by the study. The authors reported that both modalities were inaccurate for T staging (46.3% correctly staged for CT, 38.3% for ERUS), with high rates of both over- and understaging.

Considering all the evidence above together in a narrative fashion, the evidence seems to consistently support the conclusion that no significant difference exists in accuracy across CT, ERUS, and MRI for interim rectal T staging. The the level of study limitations was medium, the evidence was consistent and direct. However, a quantitative analysis cannot be done and the precision cannot be measured; therefore, the strength of evidence is low.

Interim Rectal Nodal Restaging

We identified three studies of interim rectal N restaging (summarized in Table 22). One study compared CT with ERUS, and two studies compared MRI, CT, and ERUS.

Table 22. Interim rectal N restaging

Study	Compares	Number of Patients	Design	Risk of Bias
Huh et al. 2008[164]	CT to ERUS	83 with locally advanced rectal cancer within 7 cm of anal verge	Retrospective cohort	Low
Martellucci et al. 2012[199]	CT to ERUS to MRI	37 with locally advanced rectal cancer	Prospective cohort	Moderate
Pomerri et al. 2011[163]	CT to ERUS to MRI	90 with primary rectal cancer	Prospective cohort	Low

CT=Computed tomography; ERUS=endorectal ultrasound; MRI=magnetic resonance imaging.

Huh et al. compared CT with ERUS for restaging locally advanced cancer after neoadjuvant radiochemotherapy. See Appendix C for the data reported by the study. The authors reported that CT was more sensitive than ERUS (56% vs. 50%, respectively) for detecting affected lymph nodes, but CT had a lower specificity than ERUS (74.5% vs. 81.1%, respectively). The authors concluded that neither modality was good for restaging rectal cancer.

The two studies comparing CT, MRI, and ERUS reported data sufficiently differently that only the accuracy data could be pooled quantitatively in a random-effects meta-analysis. See Appendix C for the data reported by these two studies. See Appendix D for the results of the meta-analysis. There were no statistically significant differences across the modalities, but there was a nonsignificant trend for ERUS to be more accurate than MRI and CT, and MRI to be more accurate than CT.

Two of the studies (Huh et al. and Pomerri et al.) concluded that there was no significant difference across modalities, and the third concluded that ERUS was more accurate. Our meta-analysis found a trend towards ERUS being more accurate. To explore the inconsistency further, we have summarized characteristics of the studies, patients, and imaging details that may explain the different results in Table 23, below. There is no obvious reason for the discrepancy, but the study that found ERUS to be more accurate had very low accuracies for MRI and CT compared with the two studies that considered them all approximately equal; in comparison, the reported accuracy for ERUS was similar across studies.

Table 23. Details of studies of interim rectal N restaging

tudy	Design	Patients	CT Methods	MRI Methods	ERUS Methods
Huh et al. 2008[164]	Retrospective, university-based, in Korea; mean 46 days between treatment and restaging	Locally advanced cancer near anal verge, mean age 54, 63% male	Rectal contrast, 2 readers in consensus, 70.4% accuracy	Not done	360 rotating, 7.5 or 10 MHz, 1 highly experienced reader, 72.6% accuracy
Martellucci et al. 2012[199]	Prospective, university-based, in Italy; 30–60 days between treatment and restaging	Locally advanced cancer, mean 65.5 years, 73% male	No information reported other than 3 readers in consensus, 56.5% accuracy	No information reported other than 3 readers in consensus, 55% accuracy	Enema before examination, 1 highly experienced reader, 75.5% accuracy
Pomerri et al. 2011[163]	Prospective, university-based, in Italy; 30 days between treatment and restaging	Primary rectal, median age 61, 61% male	IV contrast, 3 readers in consensus, 62% accuracy	IV contrast, enema, 1 T magnet, T1- and T2-weighted, phased-array surface coil, 3 readers in consensus, 68% accuracy	Enema before examination, rotating radial 5 to 10 MHz, 1 reader, 65% accuracy

CT=Computed tomography; ERUS=endorectal ultrasound; IV=intravenous; MRI=magnetic resonance imaging.

Considering the evidence base as a whole, the level of study limitations is medium. The evidence is somewhat inconsistent; the results of the meta-analysis are imprecise (wide confidence intervals); and the conclusion is unclear. We cannot determine whether there is significant difference across modalities or whether ERUS is slightly more accurate. Therefore, we grade the evidence as insufficient to support a conclusion as to which modality is more accurate.

Interim Rectal Metastasis Restaging
No studies that met the inclusion criteria reported on interim rectal M restaging.

Interim Rectal Circumferential Margin Status Restaging
We identified one study that reported on interim rectal CRM status. Pomerri et al.[163] conducted a prospective comparison of MRI and CT on 86 patients. The MRI was performed on a 1 Tesla machine, T1- and T2-weighted with a phased-array coil and with IV contrast agents. CT was also conducted with IV contrast material. See Appendix C for details on the reported data. MRI was more accurate than CT (85% vs. 71%, respectively) and more specific (88% vs. 74%, respectively). The authors concluded MRI can accurately identify a tumor-free CRM after neoadjuvant therapy. Although the study was rated as being at low risk of bias, a single study is insufficient to support an evidence-based conclusion.

Interim Colon Restaging
No studies that met the inclusion criteria reported on interim colon cancer restaging separately (namely, without mixing rectal cancer cases into the enrolled group).

Interim Colorectal Tumor and Nodal Restaging
No studies that met the inclusion criteria reported on interim colorectal T and N restaging.

Interim Colorectal Metastasis Restaging
We identified four studies of interim colorectal M restaging (summarized in Table 24). Three compared MRI with CT, and one compared PET/CT with CT. The study that compared PET/CT with CT reported that CT had a higher sensitivity (65.3% for CT vs. 49% for PET/CT) but a lower specificity (75% for CT vs. 83.3% for PET/CT) for detecting colorectal liver metastases. See Appendix C for the reported data. Because only one study compared PET/CT to CT, we graded the evidence as insufficient to support an evidence-based conclusion.

Table 24. Interim colorectal M restaging

Study	Compares	Number of Patients	Design	Risk of Bias
Berger-Kulemann et al. 2012[200]	CT to MRI	With fatty liver, 23	Prospective cohort	Low
Kulemann et al. 2011[201]	CT to MRI	With fatty liver, 20	Retrospective cohort	Moderate
van Kessel et al. 2011[202]	CT to MRI	20	Prospective cohort	Moderate
Lubezky et al. 2007[91]	CT to PET/CT	48	Cohort	Moderate

CT=Computed tomography; MRI=magnetic resonance imaging; PET/CT=positron emission tomography/computed tomography.

We pooled the data reported by the three studies of MRI compared with CT for detecting liver metastases. The results indicated a nonsignificant trend toward MRI being more accurate at detecting colorectal liver metastases than CT, but there was considerable heterogeneity in the data (I^2=85%). Because the data are inconsistent, we graded the evidence as insufficient to support a conclusion.

Comparative and Additive Impact of Imaging Modalities on Stage Reclassification and Management

Key Question 2b. What is the impact of alternative imaging techniques on intermediate outcomes, including stage reclassification and changes in therapeutic management?

No studies that met the inclusion criteria addressed this question.

Comparative and Additive Impact of Imaging Modalities on Clinical Outcomes

Key Question 2c. What is the impact of alternative imaging techniques on clinical outcomes?

No studies that met the inclusion criteria addressed this question.

Adverse Effects Associated With Imaging Techniques

Key Question 2d. What are the adverse effects or harms associated with using imaging techniques, including harms of test-directed management?

See the answer to Key Question 1d for harms associated with any use of these imaging tests.

Factors Affecting Accuracy

Key Question 2e. How is the comparative effectiveness of imaging techniques modified by the following factors: patient-level characteristics (e.g., age, sex, body mass index); disease characteristics (e.g., tumor grade); and imaging technique or protocol characteristics (e.g., use of different tracers or contrast agents, radiation dose of the imaging modality, slice thickness, timing of contrast)?

Two studies of MRI reported on factors affecting interim restaging accuracy. Lambregts et al.[203] performed MRI using T2 and diffusion weighted imaging after neoadjuvant chemotherapy for rectal cancer. The authors reported that diffusion-weighted MRI was unable to identify malignant lymph nodes. The other study, Macera et al.,[204] used MRI to detect liver metastases after neoadjuvant chemotherapy and concluded that a combination of contrast-enhanced T2 and diffusion-weighted MRI was more accurate than either modality in isolation. See Appendix C for more details. Because only one study reported information, the evidence base was graded as insufficient to support an evidence-based conclusion.

Conclusions for Key Question 2

We attempted to address Key Question 2.a. using systematic reviews but identified only one high-quality review of interim restaging that studied CT, MRI, and PET/CT for detecting colorectal liver metastases. MRI had a higher sensitivity for this purpose than the other modalities, but its sensitivity was probably too low in this setting to be considered clinically useful (69.9%, 95% CI: 65.6 to 73.9%).

We found that there was no significant difference in accuracy across ERUS, CT, and MRI for **interim rectal T-staging** and that there was a nonsignificant trend for MRI to be more accurate than CT for detecting **colorectal liver metastases** during restaging.

The primary conclusion to be reached for Key Question 2 is that there are gaps in the research that has been published. The evidence base is small and limited. Nine studies addressed Key Question 2. The studies were all rated as being at moderate or low risk of bias. The risk of bias ratings are provided in Appendix D. Too few studies exist to allow assessment of the possibility of publication bias using either visual analysis of funnel plots or statistical methods.

Discussion

Key Findings and Strength of Evidence

We compiled data from recent, high-quality systematic reviews to estimate the accuracy of each imaging modality in isolation. These data are summarized in Table 25. Because there were insufficient data on positron emission tomography/computed tomography (PET/CT) from systematic reviews, we examined the studies of PET/CT included in this report to address the comparative questions to estimate accuracy. An additional systematic review, Gall et al.,[84] studied only one type of endorectal probe, so due to concerns about generalizability we have not included that data in the summary table below but discuss it in the relevant section of the text.

Table 25. Accuracy of imaging tests in isolation as reported by recent systematic reviews

Staging	ERUS	CT	MRI	PET/CT
Rectal T	For identifying T1: Sensitivity: 87.8% (85.3 to 90.0%) Specificity: 98.3% (97.8 to 98.7%) For identifying T2: Sensitivity: 80.5% (77.9 to 82.9%) Specificity: 95.6% (94.9 to 96.3%) For identifying T3: Sensitivity: 96.4% (95.4 to 97.2%) Specificity: 90.6% (89.5 to 91.7%) For identifying T4: Sensitivity: 95.4% (92.4 to 97.5%) Specificity: 98.3% (97.8 to 98.7%)	For distinguishing T1/T2 from T3/T4: Sensitivity: 86% (78 to 92%) Specificity: 78% (71 to 84%)	For distinguishing T1/T2 from T3/T4: Sensitivity: 87% (81 to 92%) Specificity: 75% (68 to 80%) For identifying affected CRM: Sensitivity: 77% (57 to 90%) Specificity: 94% (88 to 97%)	Not reported
Rectal N	For identifying affected nodes: Sensitivity: 73.2% (70.6 to 75.6%) Specificity: 75.8% (73.5 to 78.0%)	For identifying affected nodes: Sensitivity: 70% (59 to 80%) Specificity: 78% (66 to 86%)	For identifying affected nodes: Sensitivity: 77% (69 to 84%) Specificity: 71% (59 to 81%)	For identifying affected nodes: Sensitivity: 61% Specificity: 83%
Colorectal T	Not reported	Not reported	Not reported	Accuracy: 95.0%
Colorectal N	Not reported	Not reported	Not reported	For identifying affected nodes: Sensitivity: 34.3% Specificity: 100%
Colorectal M	Not reported	For identifying liver metastases: Sensitivity 83.6%	For identifying liver metastases: Sensitivity: 88.2%	For identifying liver metastases: Sensitivity: 72% to 97.9%
Interim restaging	Not reported	For identifying liver metastases: Sensitivity 54% (46.7 to 62.1%)	For identifying liver metastases: Sensitivity 69.9% (65.6 to 73.9%)	For identifying liver metastases: Sensitivity 51.7% (37.8 to 65.4%)

CT=Computed tomography; ERUS=endorectal ultrasound; M=metastases stage; MRI=magnetic resonance imaging; N=nodal stage; PET=positron emission tomography; T=tumor stage. ( ) denotes the 95% confidence intervals

Our major conclusions about comparative effectiveness are listed in Table 26.

Table 26. Summary of major conclusions

Conclusion Statement	# Studies (# patients) and Study Limitations	Consistency	Directness	Precision	Strength of Evidence
ERUS is more accurate (less likely to give an incorrect result) (OR=0.36, 95% CI, 0.24 to 0.54), less likely to understage (OR=0.63, 95% CI, 0.44 to 0.89), and less likely to overstage (OR=0.47; 95% CI, 0.28 to 0.80) rectal cancer than CT in the **preoperative T staging** setting.[a]	13 studies, total N=595 Medium	Consistent	Direct	Imprecise	Low
There is no statistically significant difference in accuracy between MRI and ERUS for **preoperative rectal T staging**.	6 studies, total N=294 Medium	Consistent	Direct	Imprecise	Low
There is no statistically significant difference in accuracy across CT, MRI, or ERUS for **preoperative rectal N staging**.	18 studies, total N=845 Medium	Consistent	Direct	Imprecise	Low
While there is no statistically significant difference in accuracy between CT and MRI for **rectal N staging**, MRI is less likely to **overstage**.	4 studies, total N = 123 Medium	Consistent	Direct	Imprecise	Low
MRI is superior to CT in detecting colorectal **liver metastases** in the preoperative setting (OR=1.334; 95% CI, 1.012 to 1.761).[b]	5 studies, total N=217 Low	Consistent	Direct	Imprecise	Moderate
There is no statistically significant difference in accuracy across MRI, CT, or ERUS for **rectal T staging** in the **interim restaging** setting.	4 studies, total N=225 Medium	Consistent	Direct	Imprecise	Low
The evidence was insufficient for assessing the comparison of PET/CT to CT or MRI for **M staging or restaging**.	4 studies, total N=641; 1 study, total N=48	Inconsistent	Direct	Imprecise	Insufficient

CI=Confidence interval; CT=computed tomography; ERUS=endorectal ultrasound; IV=intravenous; M=distant metastasis stage; MRI=magnetic resonance imaging; N=nodal stage; OR=odds ratio; T=tumor stage #=number.
[a] OR < 1 indicates a lower risk of error in the first imaging modality listed in the column header; OR > 1 indicates a higher risk of error in the first imaging modality listed in the column header (with the exception of detection of liver metastases. See below)
[b] This OR > 1 indicates that MRI is more likely to deteict liver metastases than is CT.

All four imaging modalities appear to be reasonably safe. For endorectal ultrasound (ERUS), the most common adverse event appears to be pain and minor bleeding; in theory, the major adverse event of bowel perforation could occur, but no included studies reported such an event had ever occurred. Our supplementary harms searches identified a narrative review of complications of endoscopic ultrasound, including ERUS.[17] The authors noted that only one case had been reported in a prospective registry of the German Society of Ultrasound in Medicine, but did not report the number of ERUS procedures in the registry.

Harms from MRI appear to be limited to contrast agent reactions. Many of the included studies did not use intravenous contrast, and the available data suggests that the use of intravenous contrast does not improve the accuracy of MRI for rectal T or N colorectal staging.

Harms from CT include contrast agent reactions and radiation exposure. Many included studies did not use intravenous contrast, and one study suggests that using intravenous contrast does not improve CT's accuracy for rectal T or N staging.

The major harm from PET/CT is radiation exposure. A single PET/CT examination exposes the patient to about 18 mSv. Some experts believe this is a significant exposure; however, in 2010, the Health Physics Society published a position statement recommending against quantitative estimates of health risks below an individual dose of 5 rem per year (approximately 50 mSv) or a lifetime dose of 10 rem in addition to natural background radiation.[18] However, if a patient undergoes a PET/CT scan for staging, has surgical treatment, and then has regular CT scans for surveillance, the accumulated radiation dose could approach or exceed the 5 rem limit.

Indirect harms of imaging consist primarily of harms related to incorrect treatment decisions based on inaccurate staging.

Findings in Relationship to What Is Already Known

We identified a number of systematic reviews whose authors included studies reporting the accuracy of individual imaging modalities, synthesized the data for each imaging modality, and compared these summary accuracies across studies (i.e., making indirect comparisons). Bipat et al. published a systematic review in 2004 comparing the accuracy of pretreatment staging of rectal cancer by ERUS, computed tomography (CT), or magnetic resonance imaging (MRI).[205] The review authors concluded that ERUS was the most accurate modality for pretreatment rectal T staging. This finding contrasts with our finding of no statistically significant difference in accuracy of MRI and ERUS in studies that made direct comparisons. The apparent discrepancy may be because most studies in the 2004 review used older, less accurate MRI machines. It may also be due to the presence of publication bias; as indicated previously, Harewood et al. and Puli et al. both noted that the reported accuracy of ERUS declined significantly over time, and that there is evidence of publication bias in the ERUS-specific literature published before 2003.[13,14] At least one of the peer reviewers for this report noted the belief that ERUS is superior for assessing the extent of early T stage tumors, while MRI is better for assessing the extent of later T-stage tumors, but we were unable to confirm this using the included studies. The review by Bipat et al. agrees with our conclusion that ERUS was superior to CT for pretreatment rectal T staging.[205]

Lahaye et al. published a systematic review in 2005 comparing the accuracy of pretreatment N staging rectal cancer by ERUS, CT, or MRI,[206] including 84 articles. The review authors concluded that for pretreatment N staging of rectal cancer, ERUS is slightly better than MRI or CT. However, we identified no statistically significant difference across modalities for this purpose and speculate that publication bias in the early ERUS literature may have also affected Lahaye et al.'s result.

Lahaye et al. also looked at the accuracy of assessing the circumferential resection margin and included seven studies on that topic, concluding that "MRI is the only modality that predicts the circumferential resection margin with good accuracy."[206] We identified only one direct comparison study on assessing the circumferential resection margin preoperatively. In this study of 42 patients, Taylor et al. concluded that both CT and MRI tended to overstage CRM status; however, they rarely understaged CRM status.[119]

Niekel et al. published a systematic review in 2010, comparing the accuracy of pretreatment staging of colorectal liver metastases by CT, MRI, PET, or PET/CT.[15] The review authors concluded that "MR imaging is the preferred first-line modality for evaluating colorectal liver metastases in patients who have not previously undergone therapy." We did not identify any PET/CT studies that met our inclusion criteria for comparative studies, but we did find that MRI was more accurate than CT for detecting liver metastases.

Skandarajah and Tjandra published a systematic review in 2006 comparing the accuracy of pretreatment T and N staging of rectal cancer by MRI or ERUS,[207] including 31 studies of ultrasound and 8 of MRI. They concluded that ERUS and MRI are complementary and are most accurate for early localized cancers and more advanced cancers, respectively."

Kwok et al. published a systematic review in 2000, comparing the accuracy of pretreatment staging of rectal cancer by CT, MRI, or ERUS, including 83 studies, and concluding: "MRI with an endorectal coil is the single investigation that most accurately predicts pathological stage in rectal cancer."[208] Endorectal coils have since been abandoned in favor of phased-array surface coils.

The key findings from our review are summarized above, in Table 25 and Table 26. Our findings, derived from studies performing direct comparisons between modalities, seem to be in contradiction to some of the findings from systematic reviews evaluating test performance in isolation.

For example, if one compares across the prior systematic reviews it seems MRI and CT are approximately equal in accuracy, and ERUS is slightly better than either for rectal tumor stage (T) staging; however, we found that MRI and ERUS are approximately equal in accuracy and ERUS is superior to CT (see Appendix D).

A similar situation exists for rectal nodal stage (N) staging. Our analyses found that all modalities had sensitivities for detecting affected lymph nodes in the 40 percent to 50 percent range, whereas all the estimates from earlier systematic reviews found sensitivities at the 70 percent level.

We are unsure of the reason for the differences. It is true that because we included only studies that directly compared modalities that our analysis is examining a different evidence base than systematic reviews that looked at modalities in isolation. Such differences in results have been discussed in a previously published EPC methodology study.[209]

It also may be that the noncomparative ERUS and CT literature is affected by publication bias. Puli et al. concluded that there was no evidence of publication bias in the ERUS literature in 2009; however, a systematic review published in 2005 (thus, not included to address the key questions) concluded that "the performance of EUS [endoscopic ultrasound] in staging rectal cancer may be overestimated in the literature due to publication bias."[13] The review included 41 studies published between 1985 and 2003. The author, Harewood, performed visual analyses of funnel diagrams and other plots, concluding that there were few smaller studies with lower accuracy rates and that the reported accuracy appeared to be declining over time. Studies published in the surgical literature reported higher accuracies than studies published in other types of journals.[13]

Puli et al. also analyzed the reported accuracy of endoscopic ultrasound over time and found that the reported accuracy had declined significantly from the 1980s through 2000 and had stabilized or only declined slightly since then.[14] Dighe et al. reported that for N staging with CT, evidence existed that smaller studies were reporting higher accuracies (suggesting publication bias), and there was a nonsignificant trend showing the same result for T staging.[16]

Therefore, it is possible that the estimates of test accuracy for the modalities in isolation may be high due to publication bias in the noncomparative literature. We suggest focusing on the comparative-effectiveness conclusions in Table 25 instead of making indirect comparisons across the estimates of accuracy in Table 26. We derived our estimates of comparative effectiveness from direct comparisons on the same patients which are less prone to bias than indirect comparisons across different studies.

Applicability

We judged the applicability of the evidence based on the PICO framework (patients, interventions, comparisons, outcomes and settings). The majority of studies reported very little information about patient characteristics. The mean age for patients in most studies was early 60's, with a range from age 20 to as high as 93. Given that 90% of patients with rectal cancer are over age 50, the patients in these studies may be somewhat younger than is typical.

We do have some concerns about applicability with respect to the interventions. Many older studies that may have used technology that is now obsolete. For example, some of the included older MRI studies utilized devices with very low strength magnets by today's standards. Although we concurred with our Technical Expert Panel (TEP) that it did not make sense to set an arbitrary date cut-off for including studies, we did not make an a priori decision about magnet strength for MRI examinations. In addition, ERUS is an operator-dependent test, which may have to be considered when deciding whether to apply our findings in specific settings.

The EPC Methods Guide for medical tests recommends considering the following categories of outcomes in the assessment of diagnostic and prognostic tests: clinical management; direct health effects; emotional, social, cognitive and behavioral responses; legal and ethical; costs.[9] The majority of studies in this review reported only test performance outcomes. Only six studies reported changes in management based on test findings. We did not identify information on the impact of testing on emotional, social, cognitive and behavioral responses. We identified information on harms as a result of testing, but to do so, we conducted supplemental searches specifically focused on harms. We did not identify studies reporting health outcomes that resulted from treatment decisions guided by imaging test results.

We also note that most of the studies were set in university-based academic or teaching hospitals, which may limit the applicability of the results to community-based general hospitals. The majority (58%) of included primary studies were conducted in Europe, 27% in Asia and Australia, 6% in the Middle East and 9% in the United States. As we discuss in the next section, there are differences in utilization of imaging studies in the United States as compared to other countries, but we doubt that this would affect the applicability of the test performance results, assuming comparable imaging devices are utilized.

Implications for Clinical and Policy Decisionmaking

The EPC that performed the topic-refinement phase of this project noted that some stakeholders expressed interest in patterns of care and access to imaging technology for colorectal staging. Therefore, although we did not search systematically for information on this topic, we obtained relevant articles identified through our searches. Recent (2009 or later) published articles were selected for discussion.

Fourteen articles addressed patterns of care for staging of rectal cancer,[210-216] colon cancer,[217,218] colorectal cancer,[219-222] and metastases.[223]

The majority of the studies discussed using multiple imaging modalities for preoperative staging. Two studies focused only on MRI,[216,221] whereas information on PET/CT was limited.[213,223] Studies were conducted in Belgium,[210] Brazil,[214] Canada,[220] Italy,[213] the Netherlands,[221-223] New Zealand,[218] Poland,[215] Thailand,[211] and the United States.[217,219] One study was conducted in 173 U.S. and non-U.S. locations,[212] and one study was conducted in Australia and New Zealand.[216] See Appendix C for details.

To determine preoperative management of rectal cancer worldwide, Augestad et al.[212] surveyed colorectal surgeons at 173 international colorectal cancer centers from 28 countries in Africa, Asia, Europe, North America, and South America. A majority of responders were located in university hospitals (78%) and had more than 11 years' experience with rectal cancer surgery (70%). Results from 123 (71%) respondents indicated significantly more U.S. surgeons use ERUS for all patients than do non-U.S. surgeons (43.6% vs. 21.1%, respectively; statistically significant); whereas significantly fewer U.S. surgeons use MRI for all patients than do non-U.S. surgeons (20.5% vs. 42.2%, respectively; statistically significant); and similar rates were found for use of CT for all patients (56.4% by U.S. surgeons vs. 53.5% by non-U.S. surgeons; not significant [NS]).[212] The decision to use MRI was significantly influenced by multidisciplinary team meetings (relative risk [RR] 3.62, confidence interval 0.93 to 14.03; statistically significant). The authors speculated that low rates for MRI use (50% use in selected cases, 11% never use) may indicate the slow implementation of evidence-based medicine by colorectal surgeons.[212]

On a narrower geographic level, survey results from 108 members of the Colorectal Surgical Society of Australia & New Zealand indicated that 86.1 percent routinely used MRI preoperatively for suspected T2 rectal cancer, while 13.9 percent used it selectively for tumors in the lower two-thirds of the rectum.[216] The study authors noted the need for closer compliance with evidence-based guidelines in managing locally advanced rectal cancer.[216]

Ninety percent of colorectal surgeons from multidisciplinary teams and advanced facilities surveyed in Thailand routinely used CT or MRI (rectal) while 7.5 percent routinely used ERUS (middle and lower rectal) for preoperative staging. Limited availability of ERUS was noted as the cause of limited use.[211]

Lastly, a review of records from 709 patients with rectal cancer (about 70% stage III/IV) treated from 2008 to 2009 in Poland indicated that preoperative staging was performed by CT (48.1%), ERUS (23.7%), and MRI (2.5%).[215] Note that our review of the evidence indicates that CT is less accurate than ERUS for this use.

For interim staging of rectal cancer, studies conducted in Brazil[214] and Belgium[210] indicated that CT[214] or contrast-enhanced CT[210] were generally the first modality of choice. However, Brazilian surgeons and medical oncologists with more than 10 cases of rectal cancer per year preferred MRI or ERUS for local staging,[214] whereas specialized centers in Belgium preferred ERUS.[210] In Italy, ERUS (T1 and T2) and CT (T3 and T4) were chosen for distal rectal staging with single modalities, whereas CT and ERUS (T1 through T3) and CT and MRI (T4) were chosen for interim staging with combination modalities by members of the Italian Society of Surgery.[213] No studies discussed patterns of interim staging for colon cancer.

Studies discussing patients with only colon cancer (i.e., not combined with patients with rectal cancer) were not identified for inclusion in our review. However, we did identify two studies that discussed patterns of care for colon cancer.[217,218] O'Grady et al. of Fox Chase Cancer Center Partners[217] reviewed records of 124 U.S. patients given a diagnosis of stage III colon cancer (between 2003 and 2006) to determine compliance with May 2006 National Comprehensive Cancer Network (NCCN) guidelines. Compliance of staging with NCCN guidelines was 98 percent. A population-based audit of the New Zealand Cancer Registry (642 patients)[218] concluded that CT staging increased considerably from 1996 to 2003 (from 11% to 62%) while use of ultrasound remained stable.

Four studies focused on staging of colorectal cancer;[219-222] one study focused on use of MRI only.[221] In 2012, Levine et al.[219] noted that a significantly higher proportion of 288 U.S. patients with colorectal cancer referred to a multidisciplinary colorectal tumor clinic than patients treated outside the clinic underwent preoperative evaluation (as recommended by NCCN guidelines) with abdominal CT (97.5% vs. 83.1%, respectively; statistically significant), chest CT (95% vs. 37.1%, respectively; p<0.0001) and ERUS for rectal cancer (88% vs. 37.7%, respectively; statistically significant). Results from a multivariate analysis of 392 patients in Nova Scotia, Canada[220] indicated that the presence of a rectal tumor (RR 4.4, statistically significant), treatment in a community hospital (RR 1.9; statistically significant), and higher TNM staging (not statistically significant) were associated with undergoing preoperative imaging (53.1% ultimately did). Results also indicated that preoperative staging imaging (liver, pelvis), in turn, was associated with a reduced likelihood of meeting a 4-week benchmark from diagnosis-to-surgery (RR 1.0, not statistically significant). Factors such as length of waiting lists, inpatient bed availability, and mechanisms for preoperative assessment by anesthesia specialists may also have delayed surgical bookings between February 2002 and February 2004.[220]

Two population-based audits of cancer registries were conducted in the Netherlands (n=2,719).[221,222] One study noted a statistically significant increase in use of MRI for preoperative staging from 2006 to 2008 for patients with rectal cancer (73% to 85%, statistically significant)[221] The other study noted staging by abdominal ultrasound and thoracic radiography (colorectal) was being replaced by abdominal CT (colorectal) and pelvic CT or MRI (rectal) in 2005.[222]

To determine the modality of choice for evaluating metastases, Bipat et al.[223] surveyed nuclear medicine physicists, abdominal surgeons, and abdominal radiologists in the Netherlands. CT was the dominant imaging modality for staging metastases (liver, lung, and extrahepatic) despite recommendations by Dutch guidelines to use CT or MRI as a first choice for liver staging. The three most common factors affecting choice of imaging modality by specialists (surgeons and medical oncologists) were evidence in the literature, availability, and expertise. The authors also noted that Dutch guidelines lagged U.S. guidelines, in which PET/CT plays a prominent role.[223]

For changes in patient management, Melotti et al. noted that 55.6 percent of Italian surgeons surveyed believe that ^{18}F-fluorodeoxyglucose (FDG) PET/CT is incapable of modifying rectal staging either before or after chemoradiotherapy compared with other imaging modalities. This opinion, they indicate, differs from most international authors who conclude that "in 31-38 percent of patients FDG PET-CT modifies rectal staging and therefore treatment in 14-27 percent of cases."[213] No studies in our review evaluated the use of PET/CT for interim restaging of rectal cancer, but two studies that met the inclusion criteria reported the impact of adding PET/CT results to CT results for preoperative staging of colorectal cancer. The results of these studies indicate that the addition of PET/CT results did lead to changes in management, but these changes were appropriate in only half of the patients.

Limitations of the Comparative Effectiveness Review Process

Impact of Key Assumptions

The major assumption we made—that the reference standard was 100 percent accurate—is unlikely to actually be true. In most of the studies, the reference standard was intraoperative findings and histopathologic examination of tissues removed during surgery. This standard is probably close to being 100 percent accurate, but errors may occur at a low rate. For example, if a patient staged by MRI as having affected lymph nodes is staged by ERUS as not having affected lymph nodes, but has affected lymph nodes that are overlooked during surgery, ERUS would incorrectly be declared "correct." Errors in the reference standard will, presumably, result in random "noise" in the estimates of comparative effectiveness, widening the confidence intervals around the estimates. We are unaware of any work that has been able to estimate the accuracy of intraoperative findings for staging colorectal cancer.

Decisions Related to Project Scope

In an effort to keep the systematic review reasonable in scope, we elected to summarize previous systematic reviews to examine evidence on individual imaging tests used in staging evaluations compared to a reference standard. As recommended in the Methods Guide, we evaluated retrieved systematic reviews with a modified version of the AMSTAR checklist, and used the results to select higher quality systematic reviews for discussion. However, we recognize that the assessment is dependent on reporting quality, and may not completely reflect the quality of the actual systematic review. An updated review of the primary studies may yield different results from those reported in the separate systematic reviews.

Limitations of the Evidence Base

Very few studies reported on any outcomes other than staging accuracy. Among studies reporting only accuracy outcomes, we rarely found complete cross-classifed data (i.e., numbers of patients correctly staged, understaged and overstaged for each stage for all modalities and the reference standard).[209] Many of the studies that reported on staging accuracy were quite small and provided limited information on patient characteristics. In particular, the evidence base for Key Question 2, interim restaging, is very sparse even for staging accuracy outcomes.

A few studies reported on how imaging modalities affected patient management, but few of these reported whether management changes were deemed appropriate. No studies reported on patient-oriented outcomes such as survival and quality of life.

The development of a variety of treatment options for colorectal cancer, and particularly those for rectal cancer, such as local excision, sphincter-sparing surgery, total mesorectal excision, and neoadjuvant systemic treatment, has increased the importance of accurate preoperative staging. Decisions about appropriate treatment for each patient depend on the resectability of the tumor and the predicted risk of recurrence. A description of the anatomic spread of the tumor (e.g., its stage) is the most important factor in clinical decisionmaking.[224] If a method of staging is truly accurate, this should be reflected in better decisionmaking, which should result in better patient outcomes. For example, Hartman et al. published a decision model in 2013 testing thresholds for determining node positivity by MRI for making adjuvant treatment decisions for stage T2 rectal cancer. The authors found that the model's determination of benefits of treatment was dependent on the accuracy of primary tumor staging.[225]

The optimal study design for measuring the impact of staging method on patient outcomes is a large randomized controlled trial with long-term followup. In the absence of such trials, modeling can be used to estimate the impact of various staging methods on patient outcomes. For example, Lejeune et al. created a decision model set in the French health care system.[226] The model compared the use of CT with PET/CT in the management of metachronous liver metastases from colorectal cancer. The model predicted that using PET/CT instead of CT allowed 6.1 percent of patients to avoid exploratory surgery. There was no impact on overall survival, however.

Research Gaps

For characterizing gaps, we used the Hopkins EPC framework proposed by Robinson et al. (2011).[227] That system suggests that reviewers identify a set of important gaps and determine the most important reason for each gap. Each gap should be assigned one of the following reasons for the inability to draw conclusions:

- Insufficient or imprecise information: no studies, limited number of studies, sample sizes too small, estimate of effect is imprecise
- Information at risk of bias: inappropriate study design; major methodological limitations in studies
- Inconsistency or unknown consistency: consistency unknown (only 1 study); inconsistent results across studies
- Not the right information: results not applicable to population of interest; inadequate duration of interventions/comparisons; inadequate duration of followup; optimal/most important outcomes not addressed; results not applicable to setting of interest

The majority of the evidence gaps on the questions in this review fall into the category of insufficient information.

There is practically no literature on interim restaging of either colon or rectal cancer, and very few studies of staging of colon cancer; most of the literature identified was about rectal cancer. This likely reflects the relatively greater importance of clinical locoregional staging in rectal vs. colon cancer. Specifically, most studies of staging in colon cancer seemed to focus on looking for metastases, particularly to the liver.

Few studies examined the impact of combining different imaging modalities on pretreatment and interim staging assessments, which may provide more clinically relevant results than studies that examine the accuracy of one imaging modality in isolation. Given that patients often undergo multiple imaging studies for staging purposes, such information would be valuable.

Very few studies of PET/CT are available, which is a concern because, as noted above in "Patterns of Care," many experts appear to believe its addition to staging leads to useful changes in management. Also, its use for primary and interim clinical staging of patients is on the rise, despite the lack of convincing evidence to support its widespread adoption. We identified one study of changes in management after addition of PET/CT that concluded that only half of the changes in management triggered by PET/CT were appropriate, suggesting that using PET/CT for staging may result in significant patient harm.[19] Further study on this topic needs to be performed before any firm conclusions about the accuracy and clinical usefulness of PET/CT can be drawn.

"Not the right information" is another consideration. Insufficient information is available about changes in management triggered by imaging studies and about patient-oriented outcomes downstream of staging. Ideally, randomized controlled trials would be designed to test different staging and management strategies, capturing health outcomes that occur following treatment.

Studies of the impact of imaging on patient management decisions are potentially helpful and can be accomplished in shorter time frames than studies measuring health outcomes. However, it is critical to confirm whether the changes in management were appropriate. From the limited information in the studies in our review, it appears that such changes were not always appropriate.

Conclusions

Low-strength evidence suggests ERUS is more accurate than CT for preoperative rectal cancer T staging, and MRI is similar in accuracy to ERUS. Moderate-strength evidence suggests MRI is more likely to detect colorectal liver metastases than CT. Insufficient evidence was available to allow us reach any evidence-based conclusions about the use of PET/CT for colorectal cancer staging. Low-strength evidence suggests that CT, MRI, and ERUS are comparable for rectal cancer N staging, but all are limited in sensitivity. Low strength evidence suggests that they are also comparable for interim rectal cancer T restaging, but both sensitivity and specificity are suboptimal. Long-range harm from radiation exposure with repeat examinations is particularly of concern with PET/CT.

References

1. American Cancer Society (ACS). Cancer facts & figures 2012. Atlanta (GA): American Cancer Society (ACS); 2012. 65 p. Also available: http://www.cancer.org/acs/groups/content/@epidemiologysurveilance/documents/document/acspc-031941.pdf.

2. American Cancer Society (ACS). Colorectal cancer facts & figures 2011-2013. Atlanta (GA): American Cancer Society (ACS); 2011. 27 p. Also available: http://www.cancer.org/acs/groups/content/@epidemiologysurveilance/documents/document/acspc-028323.pdf.

3. Yabroff KR, Lund J, Kepka D, et al. Economic burden of cancer in the United States: estimates, projections, and future research. Cancer Epidemiol Biomarkers Prev. 2011 Oct;20(10):2006-14. PMID: 21980008

4. Mariotto AB, Yabroff KR, Shao Y, et al. Projections of the cost of cancer care in the United States: 2010-2020. J Natl Cancer Inst. 2011 Jan 19;103(2):117-28. PMID: 21228314

5. Screening for colorectal cancer. [internet]. Rockville (MD): United States Preventive Task Force (USPSTF); 2009 Mar [accessed 2013 Jan 23]. [2 p]. Available: http://www.uspreventiveservicestaskforce.org/uspstf/uspscolo.htm.

6. White CM, Ip S, McPheeters M, et al. Using existing systematic reviews to replace de novo processes in conducting Comparative Effectiveness Reviews. In: Methods guide for Comparative Effectiveness Reviews. Rockville (MD): Agency for Healthcare Research and Quality (AHRQ); 2009 Sep. Also available: http://effectivehealthcare.ahrq.gov/healthInfo.cfm?infotype=rr&ProcessID=60. PMID: 21433402

7. Owens DK, Lohr KN, Atkins D, et al. Grading the strength of a body of evidence when comparing medical interventions-Agency for Healthcare Research and Quality and the Effective Health Care Program. J Clin Epidemiol. 2010 May;63(5):513-23. PMID: 19595577

8. Owens D, Lohr K, Atkins D, et al. Grading the strength of a body of evidence when comparing medical interventions. In: Agency for Healthcare Research and Quality (AHRQ). Methods guide for comparative effectiveness reviews. Rockville (MD): Agency for Healthcare Research and Quality (AHRQ); 2009 Jul. Also available: http://effectivehealthcare.ahrq.gov/ehc/products/122/328/2009_0805_grading.pdf.

9. Agency for Healthcare Research and Quality. Methods Guide for Medical Test Reviews. AHRQ Publication No. 12-EHC017. Rockville, MD: Agency for Healthcare Research and Quality; June 2012. http://effectivehealthcare.ahrq.gov/ehc/products/246/558/Methods-Guide-for-Medical-Test-Reviews_Full-Guide_20120530.pdf.

10. Harbord RM, Deeks JJ, Egger M, et al. A unification of models for meta-analysis of diagnostic accuracy studies. Biostatistics. 2007 Apr;8(2):239-51. PMID: 16698768

11. STATA statistics/data analysis. MP parallel edition. College Station (TX): StataCorp; 1984-2007. Single user Stata for Windows. Also available: http://www.stata.com.

12. Zamora J, Abraira V, Muriel A, et al. Meta-DiSc: a software for meta-analysis of test accuracy data. BMC Med Res Methodol. 2006;6:31. PMID: 16836745

13. Harewood GC. Assessment of publication bias in the reporting of EUS performance in staging rectal cancer. Am J Gastroenterol. 2005 Apr;100(4):808-16. PMID: 15784023

14. Puli SR, Bechtold ML, Reddy JB, et al. How good is endoscopic ultrasound in differentiating various T stages of rectal cancer? Meta-analysis and systematic review. Ann Surg Oncol. 2009 Feb;16(2):254-65. PMID: 19018597

15. Niekel MC, Bipat S, Stoker J. Diagnostic imaging of colorectal liver metastases with CT, MR imaging, FDG PET, and/or FDG PET/CT: a meta-analysis of prospective studies including patients who have not previously undergone treatment. Radiology. 2010 Dec;257(3):674-84. PMID: 20829538

16. Dighe S, Purkayastha S, Swift I, et al. Diagnostic precision of CT in local staging of colon cancers: a meta-analysis. Clin Radiol. 2010 Sep;65(9):708-19. PMID: 20696298

17. Jenssen C, Alvarez-Sanchez MV, Napoleon B, et al. Diagnostic endoscopic ultrasonography: assessment of safety and prevention of complication. World J Gastroenterol. 2012 Sep 14;18(34):4659-76. PMID: 23002335

18. Radiation risk in perspective. Position statement of the Health Physics Society. McLean (VA): Health Physics Society; 2010 Jul. 4 p. Also available: http://hps.org/documents/radiationrisk.pdf.

19. Ramos E, Valls C, Martinez L, et al. Preoperative staging of patients with liver metastases of colorectal carcinoma. Does PET/CT really add something to multidetector CT? Ann Surg Oncol. 2011 Sep;18(9):2654-61. PMID: 21431987

20. Stewart SL, Wike JM, Kato I, et al. A population-based study of colorectal cancer histology in the United States, 1998-2001. Cancer. 2006 Sep 1;107(5 Suppl):1128-41. PMID: 16802325

21. Kelloff GJ, Schilsky RL, Alberts DS, et al. Colorectal adenomas: a prototype for the use of surrogate end points in the development of cancer prevention drugs. Clin Cancer Res. 2004 Jun 1;10(11):3908-18. Also available: http://clincancerres.aacrjournals.org/content/10/11/3908.full.pdf. PMID: 15173100

22. Schatzkin A, Freedman LS, Dawsey SM, et al. Interpreting precursor studies: what polyp trials tell us about large-bowel cancer. J Natl Cancer Inst. 1994 Jul 20;86(14):1053-7. PMID: 7802771

23. Levine JS, Ahnen DJ. Clinical practice. Adenomatous polyps of the colon. N Engl J Med. 2006 Dec 14;355(24):2551-7. PMID: 17167138

24. Cheng X, Chen VW, Steele B, et al. Subsite-specific incidence rate and stage of disease in colorectal cancer by race, gender, and age group in the United States, 1992-1997. Cancer. 2001 Nov 15;92(10):2547-54. PMID: 11745188

25. Cheng L, Eng C, Nieman LZ, et al. Trends in colorectal cancer incidence by anatomic site and disease stage in the United States from 1976 to 2005. Am J Clin Oncol. 2011 Dec;34(6):573-80. PMID: 21217399

26. Dukes CE. The classification of cancer of the rectum. J Pathol Bacteriol. 1932;35:323.

27. Astler VB, Coller FA. The prognostic significance of direct extension of carcinoma of the colon and rectum. Ann Surg. 1954 Jun;139(6):846-52. PMID: 13159135

28. Halappa VG, Villalobos CPC, Bonekamp S, et al. Rectal imaging: Part 1, high-resolution MRI of carcinoma of the rectum at 3 T. AJR Am J Roentgenol. 2012 Jul;199(1):W35-W42.

29. Valentini V, Cellini F. Management of local rectal cancer: evidence, controversies and future perspectives in radiotherapy. Colorectal Cancer. 2012 Apr;1(2):163-77.

30. Kaur H, Choi H, You YN, et al. MR imaging for preoperative evaluation of primary rectal cancer: practical considerations. Radiographics. 2012 Mar-Apr;32(2):389-409. PMID: 22411939

31. National Comprehensive Cancer Network (NCCN). NCCN clinical practice guidelines in oncology: colon cancer V3.2013 [slide set]. Fort Washington (PA): National Comprehensive Cancer Network (NCCN); 2012 Nov 26. 120 p. Also available: http://www.nccn.org/professionals/physician_gls/pdf/colon.pdf.

32. Fazel R, Krumholz HM, Wang Y, et al. Exposure to low-dose ionizing radiation from medical imaging procedures. N Engl J Med. 2009 Aug 27;361(9):849-57. PMID: 19710483

33. Cartana ET, Parvu D, Saftoiu A. Endoscopic ultrasound: current role and future perspectives in managing rectal cancer patients. J Gastrointest Liver Dis. 2011 Dec;20(4):407-13. PMID: 22187707

34. Burtin P, Rabot AF, Heresbach D, et al. Interobserver agreement in the staging of rectal cancer using endoscopic ultrasonography. Endoscopy. 1997 Sep;29(7):620-5. PMID: 9360871

35. Athanasiou A, Tardivon A, Ollivier L, et al. How to optimize breast ultrasound. Eur J Radiol. 2009 Jan;69(1):6-13. PMID: 18818037

36. Odegaard S, Nesje LB, Laerum OD, et al. High-frequency ultrasonographic imaging of the gastrointestinal wall. Expert Rev Med Devices. 2012 May;9(3):263-73. PMID: 22702257

37. Sehgal CM, Weinstein SP, Arger PH, et al. A review of breast ultrasound. J Mammary Gland Biol Neoplasia. 2006 Apr;11(2):113-23. PMID: 17082996

38. Martinoli C, Pretolesi F, Crespi G, et al. Power doppler sonography: clinical applications. Eur J Radiol. 1998 May;27 Suppl 2:S133-40. PMID: 9652513

39. Quality and safety: ultrasound accreditation. [internet]. Reston (VA): American College of Radiology (ACR); [accessed 2013 May 9]. [2 p]. Available: http://www.acr.org/Quality-Safety/Accreditation/Ultrasound.

40. Paakko E, Reinikainen H, Lindholm EL, et al. Low-field versus high-field MRI in diagnosing breast disorders. Eur Radiol. 2005 Jul;15(7):1361-8. PMID: 15711841

41. Beets-Tan RG. MRI in rectal cancer: the T stage and circumferential resection margin. Colorectal Dis. 2003 Sep;5(5):392-5. PMID: 12925068

42. Buchbender C, Heusner TA, Lauenstein TC, et al. Oncologic PET/MRI, part 1: tumors of the brain, head and neck, chest, abdomen, and pelvis. J Nucl Med. 2012 Jun;53(6):928-38. PMID: 22582048

43. de Souza NM, Kyriazi S, Sala E. Diffusion-weighted magnetic resonance imaging in pelvic cancer. Curr Med Imaging Rev. 2012 May;8(2):92-9.

44. Heywang-Kobrunner SH, Bick U, Bradley WG Jr, et al. International investigation of breast MRI: results of a multicentre study (11 sites) concerning diagnostic parameters for contrast-enhanced MRI based on 519 histopathologically correlated lesions. Eur Radiol. 2001;11(4):531-46. PMID: 11354744

45. Coulthard A, Potterton AJ. Pitfalls of breast MRI. Br J Radiol. 2000 Jun;73(870):665-71. PMID: 10911793

46. Kuhl CK, Schild HH. Dynamic image interpretation of MRI of the breast. J Magn Reson Imaging. 2000 Dec;12(6):965-74. PMID: 11105038

47. Lee CH. Problem solving MR imaging of the breast. Radiol Clin North Am. 2004 Sep;42(5):919-34. PMID: 15337425

48. Partridge SC, Heumann EJ, Hylton NM. Semi-automated analysis for MRI of breast tumors. Stud Health Technol Inform. 1999;62:259-60. PMID: 10538368

49. MedWatch. Information on Gadolinium-containing contrast agents. [internet]. Rockville (MD): U.S. Food and Drug Administration (FDA); 2009 Aug 13 [accessed 2010 Mar 17]. Available: http://www.fda.gov/Drugs/DrugSafety/PostmarketDrugSafetyInformationforPatientsandProviders/ucm142882.htm.

50. Fowler KJ, Linehan DC, Menias CO. Colorectal liver metastases: state of the art imaging. Ann Surg Oncol. 2013 Apr;20(4):1185-93. Epub 2012 Nov 1. PMID: 23115006

51. Sardanelli F, Iozzelli A, Fausto A. Contrast agents and temporal resolution in breast MR imaging. J Exp Clin Cancer Res. 2002 Sep;21(3 Suppl):69-75. PMID: 12585658

52. Knopp MV, Bourne MW, Sardanelli F, et al. Gadobenate Dimeglumine-enhanced MRI of the breast: analysis of dose response and comparison with Gadopentetate Dimeglumine. AJR Am J Roentgenol. 2003 Sep;181(3):663-76. PMID: 12933457

53. National Cancer Data Base (NCDB) [database online]. Chicago (IL): American College of Surgeons (ACS); 1996-1998. [accessed 1999 Mar 5]. Relative survival of breast cancer patients by AJCC stage of disease at diagnosis, 1985-1990 cases [table]. [3 p]. Available: http://www.facs.org/about_college/acsdept/cancer_dept/programs/ncdb/breastcancer4.html.

54. Dewhurst CE, Mortele KJ. Magnetic resonance imaging of rectal cancer. Radiol Clin North Am. 2013 Jan;51(1):121-31. PMID: 23182512

55. Brice J. Experts put MRI accreditation program to the test. Diagn Imaging. 2001 Jul;23(7):44-7, 49.

56. Quality and safety: computed tomography accreditation. [internet]. Reston (VA): American College of Radiology (ACR); [accessed 2013 May 10]. [2 p]. Available: http://www.acr.org/Quality-Safety/Accreditation/CT.

57. Fletcher JW, Djulbegovic B, Soares HP, et al. Recommendations on the use of 18F-FDG PET in oncology. J Nucl Med. 2008 Mar;49(3):480-508. PMID: 18287273

58. Rosen EL, Eubank WB, Mankoff DA. FDG PET, PET/CT, and breast cancer imaging. Radiographics. 2007 Oct;27 Suppl 1:S215-29. PMID: 18180228

59. Bergmann H, Dobrozemsky G, Minear G, et al. An inter-laboratory comparison study of image quality of PET scanners using the NEMA NU 2-2001 procedure for assessment of image quality. Phys Med Biol. 2005 May 21;50(10):2193-207. PMID: 15876661

60. McDonough MD, DePeri ER, Mincey BA. The role of positron emission tomographic imaging in breast cancer. Curr Oncol Rep. 2004 Jan;6(1):62-8. PMID: 14664763

61. Avril N, Schelling M, Dose J, et al. Utility of PET in breast cancer. Clin Positron Imaging. 1999 Oct;2(5):261-71. PMID: 14516650

62. Yutani K, Tatsumi M, Uehara T, et al. Effect of patients' being prone during FDG PET for the diagnosis of breast cancer. AJR Am J Roentgenol. 1999 Nov;173(5):1337-9. PMID: 10541114

63. Katanick SL. Fundamentals of ICANL accreditation. J Nucl Med Technol. 2005 Mar;33(1):19-23. PMID: 15731016

64. Dewhurst C, Rosen MP, Blake MA, et al. ACR appropriateness criteria pretreatment staging of colorectal cancer. J Am Coll Radiol. 2012 Nov;9(11):775-81. PMID: 23122343

65. Blake MA, McDermott S, Rosen MP, et al. ACR Appropriateness Criteria suspected liver metastases. [online publication]. Reston (VA): American College of Radiology (ACR); 2011. 9 p.

66. Chalmers I, Adams M, Dickersin K, et al. A cohort study of summary reports of controlled trials. JAMA. 1990 Mar 9;263(10):1401-5. PMID: 2304219

67. Neinstein LS. A review of Society for Adolescent Medicine abstracts and Journal of Adolescent Health Care articles. J Adolesc Health Care. 1987 Mar;8(2):198-203. PMID: 3818406

68. Dundar Y, Dodd S, Williamson P, et al. Case study of the comparison of data from conference abstracts and full-text articles in health technology assessment of rapidly evolving technologies: does it make a difference? Int J Technol Assess Health Care. 2006 Jul;22(3):288-94.

69. De Bellefeuille C, Morrison CA, Tannock IF. The fate of abstracts submitted to a cancer meeting: factors which influence presentation and subsequent publication. Ann Oncol. 1992 Mar;3(3):187-91. PMID: 1586615

70. Scherer RW, Langenberg P. Full publication of results initially presented in abstracts. In: Cochrane Library [Cochrane methodology review]. Issue 2. Oxford: Update Software; 2001 [accessed 2001 Apr 23]. [35 p]. Available: http://www.cochrane.org/index.htm.

71. Yentis SM, Campbell FA, Lerman J. Publication of abstracts presented at anaesthesia meetings. Can J Anaesth. 1993 Jul;40(7):632-4. PMID: 8403137

72. Marx WF, Cloft HJ, Do HM, et al. The fate of neuroradiologic abstracts presented at national meetings in 1993: rate of subsequent publication in peer-reviewed, indexed journals. AJNR Am J Neuroradiol. 1999 Jun-Jul;20(6):1173-7. PMID: 10445467

73. Moher D, Pham B, Klassen TP, et al. What contributions do languages other than English make on the results of meta-analyses? J Clin Epidemiol. 2000 Sep;53(9):964-72. PMID: 11004423

74. Juni P, Holenstein F, Sterne J, et al. Direction and impact of language bias in meta-analyses of controlled trials: empirical study. Int J Epidemiol. 2002 Feb;31(1):115-23. PMID: 11914306

75. Li FY, Lai MD. Colorectal cancer, one entity or three? J Zhejiang Univ Sci B. 2009 Mar;10(3):219-29. PMID: 19283877

76. Whiting P, Rutjes AW, Reitsma JB, et al. The development of QUADAS: a tool for the quality assessment of studies of diagnostic accuracy included in systematic reviews. BMC Med Res Methodol. 2003 Nov 10;3(1):25. PMID: 14606960

77. Lijmer JG, Mol BW, Heisterkamp S, et al. Empirical evidence of design-related bias in studies of diagnostic tests. JAMA. 1999 Sep 15;282(11):1061-6. PMID: 10493205

78. Whiting PF, Rutjes AW, Westwood ME, et al. QUADAS-2: a revised tool for the quality assessment of diagnostic accuracy studies. Ann Intern Med. 2011 Oct 18;155(8):529-36. PMID: 22007046

79. Treadwell JR, Tregear SJ, Reston JT, et al. A system for rating the stability and strength of medical evidence. BMC Med Res Methodol. 2006;6:52. Also available: http://www.biomedcentral.com/1471-2288/6/52. PMID: 17052350

80. Viswanathan M, Ansari MT, Berkman ND, et al. Assessing the risk of bias of individual studies in systematic reviews of health care interventions. Agency for Healthcare Research and Quality methods guide for Comparative Effectiveness Reviews [AHRQ Publication No. 12-EGC047-EF]. Rockville (MD): Agency for Healthcare Research and Quality (AHRQ); 2012 Mar. 33 p. Also available: http://www.effectivehealthcare.ahrq.gov.

81. Higgins JP, Thompson SG. Quantifying heterogeneity in a meta-analysis. Stat Med. 2002 Jun 15;21(11):1539-58. PMID: 12111919

82. Higgins JP, Thompson SG, Deeks JJ, et al. Measuring inconsistency in meta-analyses. BMJ. 2003 Sep 6;327(7414):557-60. PMID: 12958120

83. Atkins D, Chang S, Gartlehner G, et al. Assessing applicability when comparing medical interventions: Agency for Healthcare Research and Quality and the Effective Health Care Program. J Clin Epidemiol. 2011 Nov;64(11):1198-207. Epub 2011 Apr 3. PMID: 21463926

84. Gall TM, Markar SR, Jackson D, et al. Mini-probe ultrasonography for the staging of colon cancer. A systematic review and meta-analysis. Colorectal Dis. 2013 Oct 5. PMID: 24119196

85. Puli SR, Reddy JB, Bechtold ML, et al. Accuracy of endoscopic ultrasound to diagnose nodal invasion by rectal cancers: a meta-analysis and systematic review. Ann Surg Oncol. 2009 May;16(5):1255-65. PMID: 19219506

86. Al-Sukhni E, Milot L, Fruitman M, et al. Diagnostic accuracy of MRI for assessment of T category, lymph node metastases, and circumferential resection margin involvement in patients with rectal cancer: a systematic review and meta-analysis. Ann Surg Oncol. 2012 Jul;19(7):2212-23. PMID: 22271205

87. Lu YY, Chen JH, Ding HJ, et al. A systematic review and meta-analysis of pretherapeutic lymph node staging of colorectal cancer by 18F-FDG PET or PET/CT. Nucl Med Commun. 2012 Nov;33(11):1127-33. PMID: 23000829

88. Kim DJ, Kim JH, Ryu YH, et al. Nodal staging of rectal cancer: high-resolution pelvic MRI versus 18F-FDGPET/CT. J Comput Assist Tomogr. 2011 Sep-Oct;35(5):531-4. PMID: 21926843

89. Uchiyama S, Haruyama Y, Asada T, et al. Role of the standardized uptake value of 18-Fluorodeoxyglucose positron emission tomography-computed tomography in detecting the primary tumor and lymph node metastasis in colorectal cancers. Surg Today. 2012 Oct;42(10):956-61. PMID: 22711186

90. Orlacchio A, Schillaci O, Fusco N, et al. Role of PET/CT in the detection of liver metastases from colorectal cancer. Radiol Med. 2009 Jun;114(4):571-85. PMID: 19444590

91. Lubezky N, Metser U, Geva R, et al. The role and limitations of 18-fluro-2deoxy-d-glucose positron emission tomography (FDG-PET) scan and computerized tomography (CT) in restaging patients with hepatic colorectal [TRUNC]. J Gastrointest Surg. 2007 Apr;11(4):472-8. PMID: 17436132

92. Barbaro B, Savastano M, Sallustio G. Combined modality staging of low risk rectal cancer. Rays. 1995 Apr-Jun;20(2):145-55. PMID: 7480863

93. Yimei J, Ren Z, Lu X, et al. A comparison between the reference values of MRI and EUS and their usefulness to surgeons in rectal cancer. Eur Rev Med Pharmacol Sci. 2012 Dec;16(15):2069-77. PMID: 23280021

94. Halefoglu AM, Yildirim S, Avlanmis O, et al. Endorectal ultrasonography versus phased-array magnetic resonance imaging for preoperative staging of rectal cancer. World J Gastroenterol. 2008 Jun 14;14(22):3504-10. PMID: 18567078

95. Bianchi PP, Ceriani C, Rottoli M, et al. Endoscopic ultrasonography and magnetic resonance in preoperative staging of rectal cancer: comparison with histologic findings. J Gastrointest Surg. 2005 Dec;9(9):1222-7; discussion 1227-8. PMID: 16332477

96. Starck M, Bohe M, Fork FT, et al. Endoluminal ultrasound and low-field magnetic resonance imaging are superior to clinical examination in the preoperative staging of rectal cancer. Eur J Surg. 1995 Nov;161(11):841-5. PMID: 8749217

97. Thaler W, Watzka S, Martin F, et al. Preoperative staging of rectal cancer by endoluminal ultrasound vs. magnetic resonance imaging. Preliminary results of a prospective, comparative study. Dis Colon Rectum. 1994 Dec;37(12):1189-93. PMID: 7995142

98. Waizer A, Powsner E, Russo I, et al. Prospective comparative study of magnetic resonance imaging versus transrectal ultrasound for preoperative staging and follow-up of rectal cancer. Preliminary report. Dis Colon Rectum. 1991 Dec;34(12):1068-72. PMID: 1959456

99. Ju H, Xu D, Li D, et al. Comparison between endoluminal ultrasonography and spiral computerized tomography for the preoperative local staging of rectal carcinoma. Biosci Trends. 2009 Apr;3(2):73-6. PMID: 20103950

100. Kim NK, Kim MJ, Yun SH, et al. Comparative study of transrectal ultrasonography, pelvic computerized tomography, and magnetic resonance imaging in preoperative staging of rectal cancer. Dis Colon Rectum. 1999 Jun;42(6):770-5. PMID: 10378601

101. Osti MF, Padovan FS, Pirolli C, et al. Comparison between transrectal ultrasonography and computed tomography with rectal inflation of gas in preoperative staging of lower rectal cancer. Eur Radiol. 1997;7(1):26-30. PMID: 9000390

102. Ramana KN, Murthy PV, Rao KP, et al. Transrectal ultrasonography versus computed tomography in staging rectal carcinoma. Indian J Gastroenterol. 1997 Oct;16(4):142-3. PMID: 9357186

103. Goldman S, Arvidsson H, Norming U, et al. Transrectal ultrasound and computed tomography in preoperative staging of lower rectal adenocarcinoma. Gastrointest Radiol. 1991;16(3):259-63. PMID: 1879647

104. Pappalardo G, Reggio D, Frattaroli FM, et al. The value of endoluminal ultrasonography and computed tomography in the staging of rectal cancer: a preliminary study. J Surg Oncol. 1990 Apr;43(4):219-22. PMID: 2182943

105. Rotte KH, Kluhs L, Kleinau H, et al. Computed tomography and endosonography in the preoperative staging of rectal carcinoma. Eur J Radiol. 1989 Aug;9(3):187-90. PMID: 2680490

106. Waizer A, Zitron S, Ben-Baruch D, et al. Comparative study for preoperative staging of rectal cancer. Dis Colon Rectum. 1989 Jan;32(1):53-6. PMID: 2642791

107. Beynon J, Mortensen NJ, Foy DM, et al. Pre-operative assessment of local invasion in rectal cancer: digital examination, endoluminal sonography or computed tomography? Br J Surg. 1986 Dec;73(12):1015-7. PMID: 3539255

108. Kramann B, Hildebrandt U. Computed tomography versus endosonography in the staging of rectal carcinoma: a comparative study. Int J Colorectal Dis. 1986 Oct;1(4):216-8. PMID: 3298492

109. Rifkin MD, Wechsler RJ. A comparison of computed tomography and endorectal ultrasound in staging rectal cancer. Int J Colorectal Dis. 1986 Oct;1(4):219-23. PMID: 3298493

110. Rifkin MD, McGlynn ET, Marks G. Endorectal sonographic prospective staging of rectal cancer. Scand J Gastroenterol Suppl. 1986;123:99-103. PMID: 3535046

111. Romano G, de Rosa P, Vallone G, et al. Intrarectal ultrasound and computed tomography in the pre- and postoperative assessment of patients with rectal cancer. Br J Surg. 1985 Sep;72 Suppl:S117-9. PMID: 3899251

112. Matsuoka H, Nakamura A, Masaki T, et al. A prospective comparison between multidetector-row computed tomography and magnetic resonance imaging in the preoperative evaluation of rectal carcinoma. Am J Surg. 2003 Jun;185(6):556-9. PMID: 12781885

113. Guinet C, Buy JN, Ghossain MA, et al. Comparison of magnetic resonance imaging and computed tomography in the preoperative staging of rectal cancer. Arch Surg. 1990 Mar;125(3):385-8. PMID: 2306185

114. Hodgman CG, MacCarty RL, Wolff BG, et al. Preoperative staging of rectal carcinoma by computed tomography and 0.15T magnetic resonance imaging. Preliminary report. Dis Colon Rectum. 1986 Jul;29(7):446-50. PMID: 3720456

115. Blomqvist L, Holm T, Nyren S, et al. MR imaging and computed tomography in patients with rectal tumours clinically judged as locally advanced. Clin Radiol. 2002 Mar;57(3):211-8. PMID: 11952317

116. Fleshman JW, Myerson RJ, Fry RD, et al. Accuracy of transrectal ultrasound in predicting pathologic stage of rectal cancer before and after preoperative radiation therapy. Dis Colon Rectum. 1992 Sep;35(9):823-9. PMID: 1511639

117. Arii K, Takifuji K, Yokoyama S, et al. Preoperative evaluation of pelvic lateral lymph node of patients with lower rectal cancer: comparison study of MR imaging and CT in 53 patients. Langenbecks Arch Surg. 2006 Sep;391(5):449-54. PMID: 16847648

118. Milsom JW, Lavery IC, Stolfi VM, et al. The expanding utility of endoluminal ultrasonography in the management of rectal cancer. Surgery. 1992 Oct;112(4):832-40; discussion 840-1. PMID: 1411958

119. Taylor A, Slater A, Mapstone N, et al. Staging rectal cancer: MRI compared to MDCT. Abdom Imaging. 2007 May-Jun;32(3):323-7. PMID: 16967240

120. Bartolozzi C, Donati F, Cioni D, et al. Detection of colorectal liver metastases: a prospective multicenter trial comparing unenhanced MRI, MnDPDP-enhanced MRI, and spiral CT. Eur Radiol. 2004 Jan;14(1):14-20. PMID: 14730384

121. Bhattacharjya S, Bhattacharjya T, Baber S, et al. Prospective study of contrast-enhanced computed tomography, computed tomography during arterioportography, and magnetic resonance imaging for staging colorectal liver metastases for liver resection. Br J Surg. 2004 Oct;91(10):1361-9. PMID: 15376205

122. Bohm B, Voth M, Geoghegan J, et al. Impact of positron emission tomography on strategy in liver resection for primary and secondary liver tumors. J Cancer Res Clin Oncol. 2004 May;130(5):266-72. PMID: 14767761

123. Lencioni R, Donati F, Cioni D, et al. Detection of colorectal liver metastases: prospective comparison of unenhanced and Ferumoxides-enhanced magnetic resonance imaging at 1.5 T, dual-phase spiral CT, and spiral CT during arterial portography. Magn Reson Mater Phys Biol Med. 1998 Dec;7(2):76-87.

124. Strotzer M, Gmeinwieser J, Schmidt J, et al. Diagnosis of liver metastases from colorectal adenocarcinoma. Comparison of spiral-CTAP combined with intravenous contrast-enhanced spiral-CT and SPIO-enhanced MR combined with plain MR imaging. Acta Radiol. 1997 Nov;38(6):986-92. PMID: 9394654

125. Brown G, Davies S, Williams GT, et al. Effectiveness of preoperative staging in rectal cancer: digital rectal examination, endoluminal ultrasound or magnetic resonance imaging? Br J Cancer. 2004 Jul 5;91(1):23-9. PMID: 15188013

126. Wickramasinghe DP, Samarasekera DN. A comparison of endoanal ultrasound and computed tomography in staging rectal cancer and in clinical decision making - a preliminary study. Ceylon Med J. 2012 Mar;57(1):33-5. PMID: 22453708

127. Harewood GC, Wiersema MJ, Nelson H, et al. A prospective, blinded assessment of the impact of preoperative staging on the management of rectal cancer. Gastroenterology. 2002 Jul;123(1):24-32. PMID: 12105829

128. Engledow AH, Skipworth JR, Pakzad F, et al. The role of 18FDG PET/CT in the management of colorectal liver metastases. HPB. 2012 Jan;14(1):20-5. PMID: 22151447

129. Eglinton T, Luck A, Bartholomeusz D, et al. Positron-emission tomography/computed tomography (PET/CT) in the initial staging of primary rectal cancer. Colorectal Dis. 2010 Jul;12(7):667-73. PMID: 19486092

130. Kim SH, Jo EJ, Kim MY, et al. Clinical value of radiocontrast media skin tests as a prescreening and diagnostic tool in hypersensitivity reaction. Ann Allergy Asthma Immunol. 2013 Apr;110(4):258-62. PMID: 23535089

131. Kobayashi D, Takahashi O, Ueda T, et al. Risk factors for adverse reactions from contrast agents for computed tomograph. BMC Med Inform Decis Mak. 2013;13:18. PMID: 23363607

132. Davenport MS, Wang CL, Bashir MR, et al. Rate of contrast material extravasations and allergic-like reactions: effect of extrinsic warming of low-osmolality iodinated CT contrast material to 37 degrees. Radiology. 2012 Feb;262(2):475-84. PMID: 22106356

133. Kingston RJ, Young N, Sindhusake DP, et al. Study of patients with intravenous contrast extravasation on CT studies, with radiology staff and ward staff cannulation. J Med Imaging Radiat Oncol. 2012 Apr;56(2):163-7. PMID: 22498188

134. Mitchell AM, Jones AE, Tumlin JA, et al. Prospective study of the incidence of contrast-induced nephropathy among patients evaluated for pulmonary embolism by contrast-enhanced computed tomograph. Acad Emerg Med. 2012 Jun;19(6):618-25. PMID: 22687176

135. Vogl TJ, Wessling J, Buerke B. An observational study to evaluate the efficiency and safety of Ioversol pre-filled syringes compared with Ioversol bottles in contrast-enhanced examination. Acta Radiol. 2012 Oct 1;53(8):914-20. PMID: 22983259

136. Cadwallader RA, Walsh SR, Burrows B, et al. Prospective audit of cross-sectional imaging and radiation exposure in general surgical patients. Ann R Coll Surg Engl. 2011 Jan;93(1):6-8. PMID: 20955661

137. Hatakeyama S, Abe A, Suzuki T, et al. Clearance and safety of the radiocontrast medium Iopamidol in peritoneal dialysis patients. Int J Nephrol. 2011;2011:657051. PMID: 22028966

138. Loh S, Bagheri S, Katzberg RW, et al. Delayed adverse reaction to contrast-enhanced CT: a prospective single-center study comparison to control group without enhancement. Radiology. 2010 Jun;255(3):764-71. PMID: 20406882

139. Ozbulbul NI, Yurdakul M, Tola M. Comparison of a low-osmolar contrast medium, Iopamidol, and an iso-osmolar contrast medium, Iodixanol, in MDCT coronary angiography. Coron Artery Dis. 2010 Nov;21(7):414-9. PMID: 20671550

140. Shah-Patel LR, Piraner M, Silberzweig JE. Adverse events in a freestanding radiology office. J Am Coll Radiol. 2009 Apr;6(4):263-7. PMID: 19327659

141. Shie RF, Pan KT, Chu SY, et al. Immediate adverse drug reactions in computed tomography with slow injection rate: comparing Iothalamate Meglumine with Iopromide. Chin J Radiol. 2008 Dec;33(4):233-8.

142. Weisbord SD, Mor MK, Resnick AL, et al. Prevention, incidence, and outcomes of contrast-induced acute kidney injury. Arch Intern Med. 2008 Jun 23;168(12):1325-32. PMID: 18574090

143. Yang SC, Liu SH, Chang KM. Iothalamate Meglumine induced transient tachycardia during intravenous bolus injection for CT and parameters related to its discomfort. Chin J Radiol. 2008 Sep;33(3):131-6.

144. Jung KE, Chung J, Park BC, et al. A clinical study of cutaneous adverse reactions to nonionic contrast media in Korea. Ann Dermatol. 2012 Feb;24(1):22-5. PMID: 22363151

145. Cote GA, Hovis RM, Ansstas MA, et al. Incidence of sedation-related complications with Propofol use during advanced endoscopic procedures. Clin Gastroenterol Hepatol. 2010 Feb;8(2):137-42. PMID: 19607937

146. Kalaitzakis E, Varytimiadis K, Meenan J. Predicting what can go wrong at endoscopic ultrasound: a large series experience. Frontline Gastroenterol. 2011 Apr;2(2):110-6.

147. Niv Y, Gershtansky Y, Kenett RS, et al. Complications in Endoscopic Retrograde Cholangiopancreatography (ERCP) and Endoscopic Ultrasound (EUS): analysis of 7-year physician-reported adverse events. Drug Healthc Patient Saf. 2011;3:21-5. PMID: 21753900

148. Schilling D, Rosenbaum A, Schweizer S, et al. Sedation with Propofol for interventional endoscopy by trained nurses in high-risk octogenarians: a prospective, randomized, controlled study. Endoscopy. 2009 Apr;41(4):295-8. PMID: 19340730

149. Fatima H, DeWitt J, LeBlanc J, et al. Nurse-administered Propofol sedation for upper endoscopic ultrasonography. Am J Gastroenterol. 2008 Jul;103(7):1649-56. PMID: 18557709

150. Semelka RC, Hernandes Mde A, Stallings CG, et al. Objective evaluation of acute adverse events and image quality of Gadolinium-based contrast agents (Gadobutrol and Gadobenate Dimeglumine) by blinded evaluation. Pilot study. Magn Reson Imaging. 2013 Jan;31(1):96-101. PMID: 22898688

151. Albiin N, Kartalis N, Bergquist A, et al. Manganese Chloride Tetrahydrate (CMC-001) enhanced liver MRI: evaluation of efficacy and safety in healthy volunteer. MAGMA. 2012 Oct;25(5):361-8. PMID: 22399275

152. Bredart A, Kop JL, Fall M, et al. Perception of care and experience of examination in women at risk of breast cancer undergoing intensive surveillance by standard imaging with or without MR. Patient Educ Couns. 2012 Mar;86(3):405-13. PMID: 21795009

153. Maurer M, Heine O, Wolf M, et al. Tolerability and diagnostic value of Gadoteric Acid in the general population and in patients with risk factors: results in more than 84,000 patient. Eur J Radiol. 2012 May;81(5):885-90. PMID: 21555197

154. Voth M, Rosenberg M, Breuer J. Safety of Gadobutrol, a new generation of contrast agents: experience from clinical trials and postmarketing surveillance. Invest Radiol. 2011 Nov;46(11):663-71. PMID: 21623211

155. Forsting M, Palkowitsch P. Prevalence of acute adverse reactions to Gadobutrol--a highly concentrated macrocyclic gadolinium chelate: review of 14,299 patients from observational trials. Eur J Radiol. 2010 Jun;74(3):e186-92. PMID: 19574008

156. Ichikawa T, Saito K, Yoshioka N, et al. Detection and characterization of focal liver lesions: a Japanese phase III, multicenter comparison between Gadoxetic Acid Disodium-enhanced magnetic resonance imaging and contrast-enhanced computed tomography predominantly in patients with hepatocellular carcinoma and chronic liver disease. Invest Radiol. 2010 Mar;45(3):133-41. PMID: 20098330

157. Ishiguchi T, Takahashi S. Safety of Gadoterate Meglumine (Gd-DOTA) as a contrast agent for magnetic resonance imaging: results of a post-marketing surveillance study in Japan. Drugs R D. 2010;10(3):133-45. PMID: 20945944

158. Leander P, Golman K, Mansson S, et al. Orally administered Manganese with and without Ascorbic Acid as a liver-specific contrast agent and bowel marker for magnetic resonance imaging: phase I clinical trial assessing efficacy and safety. Invest Radiol. 2010 Sep;45(9):559-64. PMID: 20644487

159. Hammersting R, Adam G, Ayuso J-RA, et al. Comparison of 1.0 M Gadobutrol and 0.5 m Gadopentetate Dimeglumine-enhanced magnetic resonance imaging in five hundred seventy-two patients with known or suspected liver lesions. Invest Radiol. 2009 Mar;44(3):168-76. PMID: 19169143

160. Schieren G, Tokmak F, Lefringhausen L, et al. C-reactive protein levels and clinical symptoms following Gadolinium administration in hemodialysis patients. Am J Kidney Dis. 2008 Jun;51(6):976-86. PMID: 18501785

161. Codreanu I, Dasanu CA, Weinstein GS, et al. Fluorodeoxyglucose-induced allergic reaction: a case report. J Oncol Pharm Pract. 2013 Mar;19(1):86-8. PMID: 22267446

162. Wink MH, Wijkstra H, De La Rosette JJ, et al. Ultrasound imaging and contrast agents: a safe alternative to MRI? Minim Invasive Ther Allied Technol. 2006 Apr;15(2):93-100. PMID: 16754192

163. Pomerri F, Pucciarelli S, Maretto I, et al. Prospective assessment of imaging after preoperative chemoradiotherapy for rectal cancer. Surgery. 2011 Jan;149(1):56-64. PMID: 20452636

164. Huh JW, Park YA, Jung EJ, et al. Accuracy of endorectal ultrasonography and computed tomography for restaging rectal cancer after preoperative chemoradiation. J Am Coll Surg. 2008 Jul;207(1):7-12. PMID: 18589355

165. Mo LR, Tseng LJ, Jao YT, et al. Balloon sheath miniprobe compared to conventional EUS in the staging of colorectal cancer. Hepatogastroenterology. 2002 Jul-Aug;49(46):980-3. PMID: 12143258

166. Brenner DJ, Hall EJ. Computed tomography--an increasing source of radiation exposure. N Engl J Med. 2007 Nov 29;357(22):2277-84. PMID: 18046031

167. Fact sheet: computed tomography (CT) scans and cancer. [internet]. Bethesda (MD): National Cancer Institute (NCI); 2013 Jul 16 [accessed 2013 Jul 30]. [9 p]. Available: http://www.cancer.gov/cancertopics/factsheet/detection/CT.

168. Medical magnetic resonance (MR) procedures: protection of patients. Health Phys. 2004 Aug;87(2):197-216. PMID: 15257220

169. Shellock FG. Radiofrequency energy-induced heating during MR procedures: a review. J Magn Reson Imaging. 2000 Jul;12(1):30-6. PMID: 10931562

170. Fiek M, Remp T, Reithmann C, et al. Complete loss of ICD programmability after magnetic resonance imaging. Pacing Clin Electrophysiol. 2004 Jul;27(7):1002-4. PMID: 15271024

171. Shellock FG. Magnetic resonance safety update 2002: implants and devices. J Magn Reson Imaging. 2002 Nov;16(5):485-96. PMID: 12412025

172. Foster JR, Hall DA, Summerfield AQ, et al. Sound-level measurements and calculations of safe noise dosage during EPI at 3 T. J Magn Reson Imaging. 2000 Jul;12(1):157-63. PMID: 10931575

173. Dempsey MF, Condon B, Hadley DM. Investigation of the factors responsible for burns during MRI. J Magn Reson Imaging. 2001 Apr;13(4):627-31. PMID: 11276109

174. Feychting M. Health effects of static magnetic fields--a review of the epidemiological evidence. Prog Biophys Mol Biol. 2005 Feb-Apr;87(2-3):241-6. PMID: 15556662

175. Hong CZ, Shellock FG. Short-term exposure to a 1.5 tesla static magnetic field does not affect somato-sensory-evoked potentials in man. Magn Reson Imaging. 1990;8(1):65-9. PMID: 2325519

176. Shellock FG, Schaefer DJ, Gordon CJ. Effect of a 1.5 T static magnetic field on body temperature of man. Magn Reson Med. 1986 Aug;3(4):644-7. PMID: 3747826

177. Budinger TF. Nuclear magnetic resonance (NMR) in vivo studies: known thresholds for health effects. J Comput Assist Tomogr. 1981 Dec;5(6):800-11. PMID: 7033311

178. Chang Y, Lee GH, Kim TJ, et al. Toxicity of magnetic resonance imaging agents: small molecule and nanoparticle. Curr Top Med Chem. 2013;13(4):434-45. PMID: 23432006

179. American College of Radiology. ACR manual on contrast media [version 9]. Reston (VA): American College of Radiology; 2013. 128 p.

180. Thomsen HS. Nephrogenic systemic fibrosis. Imaging Decis. 2008 Mar 21;11(4):13-8.

181. Grobner T. Gadolinium--a specific trigger for the development of nephrogenic fibrosing dermopathy and nephrogenic systemic fibrosis. Nephrol Dial Transplant. 2006 Apr;21(4):1104-8. PMID: 16431890

182. FDA drug safety communication: new warnings for using Gadolinium-based contrast agents in patients with kidney dysfunction. [internet]. Silver Spring (MD): U.S. Food and Drug Administration (FDA); 2010 Dec 23 [accessed 2013 Jul 29]. [3 p]. Available: http://www.fda.gov/Drugs/DrugSafety/ucm223966.htm.

183. Public health advisory - Gadolinium-containing contrast agents for magnetic resonance imaging (MRI). [internet]. Silver Spring (MD): U.S. Food and Drug Administration (FDA); 2006 Jun 8 [updated 2010 Jun 22]; [accessed 2013 Jul 29]. [2 p]. Available: http://www.fda.gov/Drugs/DrugSafety/PostmarketDrugSafetyInformationforPatientsandProviders/DrugSafetyInformationforHeathcareProfessionals/PublicHealthAdvisories/ucm053112.htm.

184. FDA requests boxed warning for contrast agents used to improve MRI images. [internet]. Silver Spring (MD): U.S. Food and Drug Administration (FDA); 2007 May 23 [updated 2013 Apr 10]; [accessed 2013 Jul 29]. [2 p]. Available: http://www.fda.gov/NewsEvents/Newsroom/PressAnnouncements/2007/ucm108919.htm.

185. Cronin B, Marsden PK, O'Doherty MJ. Are restrictions to behaviour of patients required following Fluorine-18 Fluorodeoxyglucose positron emission tomographic studies? Eur J Nucl Med. 1999 Feb;26(2):121-8. PMID: 9933345

186. Kim S, Lim HK, Lee SJ, et al. Depiction and local staging of rectal tumors: comparison of transrectal US before and after water instillation. Radiology. 2004 Apr;231(1):117-22. PMID: 15068943

187. Hunerbein M, Pegios W, Rau B, et al. Prospective comparison of endorectal ultrasound, three-dimensional endorectal ultrasound, and endorectal MRI in the preoperative evaluation of rectal tumors. Preliminary results. Surg Endosc. 2000 Nov;14(11):1005-9. PMID: 11116406

188. Rafaelsen SR, Sorensen T, Jakobsen A, et al. Transrectal ultrasonography and magnetic resonance imaging in the staging of rectal cancer. Effect of experience. Scand J Gastroenterol. 2008;43(4):440-6. PMID: 18365909

189. Skriver EB, Nielsen MB, Qvitzau S, et al. Comparison of precontrast, postcontrast, and delayed CT scanning for the staging of rectal carcinoma. Gastrointest Radiol. 1992;17(3):267-70. PMID: 1612314

190. Lupo L, Angelelli G, Pannarale O, et al. Improved accuracy of computed tomography in local staging of rectal cancer using water enema. Int J Colorectal Dis. 1996;11(2):60-4. PMID: 8739828

191. Wicherts DA, de Haas RJ, van Kessel CS, et al. Incremental value of arterial and equilibrium phase compared to hepatic venous phase CT in the preoperative staging of colorectal liver metastases: an evaluation with different reference standards. Eur J Radiol. 2011 Feb;77(2):305-11. PMID: 19695807

192. Koh DM, Collins DJ, Wallace T, et al. Combining diffusion-weighted MRI with Gd-EOB-DTPA-enhanced MRI improves the detection of colorectal liver metastases. Br J Radiol. 2012 Jul;85(1015):980-9. PMID: 22167501

193. Jao SY, Yang BY, Weng HH, et al. Evaluation of Gadolinium-enhanced T1-weighted magnetic resonance imaging in the preoperative assessment of local staging in rectal cancer. Colorectal Dis. 2010 Nov;12(11):1139-48. PMID: 19548900

194. Vliegen RF, Beets GL, von Meyenfeldt MF, et al. Rectal cancer: MR imaging in local staging--is Gadolinium-based contrast material helpful? Radiology. 2005 Jan;234(1):179-88. PMID: 15550372

195. Okizuka H, Sugimura K, Yoshizako T, et al. Rectal carcinoma: prospective comparison of conventional and gadopentetate dimeglumine enhanced fat-suppressed MR imaging. J Magn Reson Imaging. 1996 May-Jun;6(3):465-71. PMID: 8724412

196. Kim MJ, Lim JS, Oh YT, et al. Preoperative MRI of rectal cancer with and without rectal water filling: an intraindividual comparison. AJR Am J Roentgenol. 2004 Jun;182(6):1469-76. PMID: 15149992

197. Futterer JJ, Yakar D, Strijk SP, et al. Preoperative 3T MR imaging of rectal cancer: local staging accuracy using a two-dimensional and three-dimensional T2-weighted turbo spin echo sequence. Eur J Radiol. 2008 Jan;65(1):66-71. PMID: 18164156

198. van Kessel CS, Buckens CF, van den Bosch MA, et al. Preoperative imaging of colorectal liver metastases after neoadjuvant chemotherapy: a meta-analysis. Ann Surg Oncol. 2012 Sep;19(9):2805-13. PMID: 22396005

199. Martellucci J, Scheiterle M, Lorenzi B, et al. Accuracy of transrectal ultrasound after preoperative radiochemotherapy compared to computed tomography and magnetic resonance in locally advanced rectal cancer. Int J Colorectal Dis. 2012 Jul;27(7):967-73. PMID: 22297865

200. Berger-Kulemann V, Schima W, Baroud S, et al. Gadoxetic acid-enhanced 3.0 T MR imaging versus multidetector-row CT in the detection of colorectal metastases in fatty liver using intraoperative ultrasound and histopathology as a standard of reference. Eur J Surg Oncol. 2012 Aug;38(8):670-6. PMID: 22652037

201. Kulemann V, Schima W, Tamandl D, et al. Preoperative detection of colorectal liver metastases in fatty liver: MDCT or MRI? Eur J Radiol. 2011 Aug;79(2):e1-6. PMID: 20392584

202. van Kessel CS, van Leeuwen MS, van den Bosch MA, et al. Accuracy of multislice liver CT and MRI for preoperative assessment of colorectal liver metastases after neoadjuvant chemotherapy. Dig Surg. 2011;28(1):36-43. PMID: 21293130

203. Lambregts DM, Maas M, Riedl RG, et al. Value of ADC measurements for nodal staging after chemoradiation in locally advanced rectal cancer-a per lesion validation study. Eur Radiol. 2011 Feb;21(2):265-73. PMID: 20730540

204. Macera A, Lario C, Petracchini M, et al. Staging of colorectal liver metastases after preoperative chemotherapy. Diffusion-weighted imaging in combination with Gd-EOB-DTPA MRI sequences increases sensitivity and diagnostic accuracy. Eur Radiol. 2013 Mar;23(3):739-47. PMID: 22976920

205. Bipat S, Glas AS, Slors FJ, et al. Rectal cancer: local staging and assessment of lymph node involvement with endoluminal US, CT, and MR imaging--a meta-analysis. Radiology. 2004 Sep;232(3):773-83. PMID: 15273331

206. Lahaye MJ, Engelen SM, Nelemans PJ, et al. Imaging for predicting the risk factors--the circumferential resection margin and nodal disease--of local recurrence in rectal cancer: a meta-analysis. Semin Ultrasound CT MR. 2005 Aug;26(4):259-68. PMID: 16152740

207. Skandarajah AR, Tjandra JJ. Preoperative loco-regional imaging in rectal cancer. ANZ J Surg. 2006 Jun;76(6):497-504. PMID: 16768778

208. Kwok H, Bissett IP, Hill GL. Preoperative staging of rectal cancer. Int J Colorectal Dis. 2000 Feb;15(1):9-20. PMID: 10766086

209. Trikalinos TA, Hoaglin DC, Small KM, et al. Evaluating practices and developing tools for comparative effectiveness reviews of diagnostic test accuracy: methods for the joint meta-analysis of multiple tests (Prepared by the Tufts Evidence-based Practice Center, under Contract No. 290 2007-10055-I.). Rockville (MD): Agency for Healthcare Research and Quality (AHRQ); 2013 Jan. 49 p. Also available: http://www.effectivehealthcare.ahrq.gov/ehc/products/291/1380/Methods%20Report_Evaluating-Practices-Developing-Tools_Final_01-14-2013.pdf.

210. Magne N, Daisne JF, Moretti L, et al. A practice survey of the evolution of rectal cancer management: a Belgian Federal College of radiotherapy study. Bull Cancer (Paris). 2009 Jul-Aug;96(7):E45-51. PMID: 19617178

211. Lohsiriwat V, Lohsiriwat D, Thavichaigarn P. Current practices in rectal cancer surgery: a survey of Thai colorectal surgeons. J Med Assoc Thai. 2009 Aug;92(8):1009-15. PMID: 19694323

212. Augestad KM, Lindsetmo RO, Stulberg J, et al. International preoperative rectal cancer management: staging, neoadjuvant treatment, and impact of multidisciplinary teams. World J Surg. 2010 Nov;34(11):2689-700. PMID: 20703471

213. Melotti G, De Antoni E, Habr-Gama A, et al. Management of distal rectal cancer: results from a national survey. Updates Surg. 2013 Mar;65(1):43-52. Epub 2013 Jan 19. PMID: 23335049

214. Habr-Gama A, Perez RO, Sao Juliao GP, et al. Factors affecting management decisions in rectal cancer in clinical practice: results from a national survey. Tech Coloproctol. 2011 Mar;15(1):45-51. PMID: 21057971

215. Mroczkowski P, Hac S, Mik M, et al. Preliminary results of the first quality assurance project in rectal cancer in Poland. Pol Przegl Chir. 2011 Mar;83(3):144-9. PMID: 22166316

216. Ooi K, Frizelle F, Ong E, et al. Current practice in preoperative therapy and surgical management of locally advanced rectal cancer: a bi-national survey. Colorectal Dis. 2012 Jul;14(7):814-20. PMID: 21899709

217. O'Grady MA, Slater E, Sigurdson ER, et al. Assessing compliance with national comprehensive cancer network guidelines for elderly patients with stage III colon cancer: the Fox Chase Cancer Center Partners' initiative. Clin Colorectal Cancer. 2011 Jun;10(2):113-6. PMID: 21859563

218. Cunningham R, Sarfati D, Hill S, et al. Colon cancer management in New Zealand: 1996-2003. N Z Med J. 2009 May 8;122(1294):51-60. PMID: 19465947

219. Levine RA, Chawla B, Bergeron S, et al. Multidisciplinary management of colorectal cancer enhances access to multimodal therapy and compliance with National Comprehensive Cancer Network (NCCN) guidelines. Int J Colorectal Dis. 2012 Nov;27(11):1531-8. PMID: 22645076

220. McConnell YJ, Inglis K, Porter GA. Timely access and quality of care in colorectal cancer: are they related? Int J Qual Health Care. 2010 Jun;22(3):219-28. PMID: 20207714

221. van der Geest LG, Krijnen P, Wouters MW, et al. Improved guideline compliance after a 3-year audit of multidisciplinary colorectal cancer care in the western part of the Netherlands. J Surg Oncol. 2012 Jul 1;106(1):1-9. PMID: 22234959

222. van Steenbergen LN, Lemmens VE, Straathof JW, et al. Improvable quality of diagnostic assessment of colorectal cancer in southern Netherlands. Eur J Gastroenterol Hepatol. 2009 May;21(5):570-5. PMID: 19190499

223. Bipat S, Niekel MC, Comans EF, et al. Imaging modalities for the staging of patients with colorectal cancer. Neth J Med. 2012 Jan;70(1):26-34. PMID: 22271811

224. Heriot AG, Grundy A, Kumar D. Preoperative staging of rectal carcinoma. Br J Surg. 1999 Jan;86(1):17-28. PMID: 10027354

225. Hartman RI, Chang CY, Wo JY, et al. Optimizing adjuvant treatment decisions for stage T2 rectal cancer based on mesorectal node size. A decision analysis. Acad Radiol. 2013 Jan;20(1):79-89.

226. Lejeune C, Bismuth MJ, Conroy T, et al. Use of a decision analysis model to assess the cost-effectiveness of 18F-FDG PET in the management of metachronous liver metastases of colorectal cancer. J Nucl Med. 2005 Dec;46(12):2020-8. PMID: 16330566

227. Robinson KA, Saldanha IJ, Mckoy NA. Frameworks for determining research gaps during systematic reviews. Rockville (MD): Agency for Healthcare Research and Quality (AHRQ); 2011 Jun. 79 p. (Methods future research needs report; no.2). Also available: http://www.effectivehealthcare.ahrq.gov/ehc/products/201/735/FRN2_Frameworks_20110726.pdf.

228. Paul MA, Visser JJ, Mulder C, et al. The use of biliary CEA measurements in the diagnosis of recurrent colorectal cancer. Eur J Surg Oncol. 1997 Oct;23(5):419-23. PMID: 9393570

229. Kim H, Lim JS, Choi JY, et al. Rectal cancer: comparison of accuracy of local-regional staging with two- and three-dimensional preoperative 3-T MR imaging. Radiology. 2010 Feb;254(2):485-92. PMID: 20093520

230. Yang L, Krefting I, Gorovets A, et al. Nephrogenic systemic fibrosis and class labeling of Gadolinium-based contrast agents by the Food and Drug Administration. Radiology. 2012 Oct;265(1):248-53. Also available: http://pubs.rsna.org/doi/pdf/10.1148/radiol.12112783. PMID: 22923714

Abbreviations and Acronyms

95% CI:	95% confidence interval
ACR:	American College of Radiology
AJCC:	American Joint Committee on Cancer
ASA:	American Society of Anesthesiologists
ASA III:	American Society of Anesthesiologists Class III
ASA IV:	American Society of Anesthesiologists Class IV
bpm:	beats per minute
CER:	comparative effectiveness review
CIAKI:	contrast-induced acute kidney injury
CINAHL:	Cumulative Index to Nursing and Allied Health Literature database
cm:	centimeter
CRM:	circumferential resection margin
CT:	computed tomography
CTPA:	computed tomography pulmonary angiography
DARE:	Database of Reviews of Effectiveness
DBE:	double-balloon endoscopy
EPC:	Evidence-based Practice Center
ERCP:	endoscopic retrograde cholangiopancreatography
ERUS:	endorectal ultrasound
EUS:	endoscopic ultrasound
FDA:	U.S. Food and Drug Administration
FDG:	^{18}F-fluorodeoxyglucose
GBCA:	gadolinium-based contrast agent
IV:	intravenous
kg:	kilogram
M:	metastases stage
MDCT:	multiphase detector computed tomography
MHz:	megahertz
mg:	milligram
ml:	milliliter
mm:	millimeter
mm Hg:	millimeters of Mercury
MRI:	magnetic resonance imaging
N:	number
N stage:	nodal stage
NR:	not reported
NS:	not significant
NY:	New York
OR:	odds ratio
PET:	positron emission tomography
PET/CT:	positron emission tomography/computed tomography
pN:	pathologic nodal stage
pT:	pathologic tumor stage
QUADAS:	quality assessment tool for diagnostic accuracy studies
SD:	standard deviation

SpO$_2$:	oxygen saturation measured by pulse oximetry
SROC:	summary receiver operating characteristic
T stage:	tumor stage
T:	Tesla
USA:	United States of America

Glossary of Selected Terms

Accuracy — Number of correctly staged cancers divided by the total number of all staged cancers.

Overstaged — Classified by the imaging modality as being of a higher stage than the stage defined by the reference standard.

Odds ratio — The odds of a staging error for a given modality is the rate of errors divided by the inverse of the rate of errors. The odds ratio is the odds of an error by one imaging modality divided by the odds of an error by another imaging modality. If the odds ratio is 1, no difference exists in odds of incorrect staging between the two modalities. If there is a difference, the odds ratio will be larger or smaller than 1 (depending on which imaging modality was selected to be the denominator, usually an arbitrary decision).

Sensitivity — The number of true positives divided by the sum of true positives and false negatives. Sensitivity is the proportion of people with the disease who have a positive test for the disease. A test with high sensitivity will rarely misclassify people with the disease as not having the disease (the test has a low rate of false negatives).

Specificity — The number of true negatives divided by the sum of true negatives and false positives. Specificity is the proportion of people without the disease who have a negative test. A test with high specificity will rarely misclassify people without the disease as diseased (a low rate of false positives).

Understaged — Classified by the imaging modality as being of a lower stage than the stage defined by the reference standard.

Appendix A. Search Strategy

Resources Searched

ECRI Institute information specialists searched the following databases for relevant information. Search terms and strategies for each resource appear below.

Table A-1. Databases searched for relevant information

Name	Date Limits	Platform/Provider
The Cochrane Central Register of Controlled Trials (CENTRAL)	1990 through February 21, 2013	Wiley
The Cochrane Database of Methodology Reviews (Methodology Reviews)	1990 through February 21, 2013	Wiley
The Cochrane Database of Systematic Reviews (Cochrane Reviews)	1990 through February 21, 2013	Wiley
Database of Abstracts of Reviews of Effects (DARE)	1990 through February 21, 2013	Wiley
EMBASE (Excerpta Medica)	1980 through October 23, 2013 for main search & 2008 through May 31, 2013 for safety search	OVIDSP
Health Technology Assessment Database (HTA)	1990 through February 21, 2013	Wiley
MEDLINE	1980 through October 23, 2013 for main search & 2008 through May 31, 2013 for safety search	OVIDSP
PubMed (PreMEDLINE)	Searched on October 23, 2013 for main search & 2008 through May 31, 2013 for safety search	NLM
U.K. National Health Service Economic Evaluation Database (NHS EED)	1990 through February 21, 2013	Wiley

Topic-Specific Search Terms

The search strategies employed combinations of free-text keywords as well as controlled vocabulary terms including (but not limited to) the following concepts. Strategies for each bibliographic database follow this table.

Table A-2. Medical Subject Headings (MeSH), EMTREE, and keywords

Concept	Controlled Vocabulary	Keywords
Cancer	*MeSH* Colorectal Neoplasms *EMTREE* Colon Cancer Colon Tumor Rectum Cancer Rectum Tumor	Adenocarcinoma$ Cancer$ Carcinoma$ Colon$ Colorectal Neoplas$ Rect$ Tumo$
Staging	*MeSH* Neoplasm Staging *EMTREE* Cancer Staging	Re-stag$ Restag$ Stag$
Imaging	*MeSH* Diagnostic Imaging Endoscopy, Gastrointestinal Magnetic Resonance Imaging Tomography, Emission-Computed Tomography, X-Ray Computed Radiography, Thoracic Ultrasonography *EMTREE* Computer Assisted Emission Tomography Computer Assisted Tomography Echography Gastrointestinal Endoscopy Positron Emission Tomography Multidetector Computed Tomography Nuclear Magnetic Resonance Imaging Thorax Radiography	Computed tomography Computerized tomography CT Endorectal Endoscop$ ERUS EUS Imag$ Magnetic resonance imaging MD-CT MRI Multidetector computerized tomography PET Positron emission tomography Transabdominal Transrectal TRUS TUS Ultrasound X-ray
Imaging Agents	*MeSH* Contrast Media *EMTREE* Contrast Medium	Agent$ Contrast Medium$
Radiation	*MeSH* Radiation Injuries *EMTREE* Radiation Injury	Injury Radiation

Table A-2. Medical Subject Headings (MeSH), EMTREE, and keywords (continued)

Concept	Controlled Vocabulary	Keywords
Harms & Adverse Events	*MeSH* Medical Errors *EMTREE* Medical Error	Adverse Effect$ Error$ Event$ Harm$ Outcome$ Reaction$

Search Strategies

Table A-3. EMBASE/MEDLINE (presented in OVID syntax)

Set #	Concept	Search Statement
1	Colorectal Cancer	exp Colorectal Neoplasms/ or exp colon cancer/ or exp colon tumor/ or exp rectum cancer/ or exp rectum tumor/ or ((Colon$ or colorectal or rect$) adj2 (cancer$ or tumo$ or neoplas$ or carcinoma$ or adenocarcinoma$)).ti,ab.
2	Staging	neoplasm staging/ or cancer staging/ or (stag$ or restag$ or re-stag$).ti,ab.
3	Imaging Controlled Vocabulary	exp Diagnostic Imaging/ or exp Tomography, Emission-Computed/ or exp Tomography, X-Ray Computed/ or exp Magnetic Resonance Imaging/ or exp Ultrasonography/ or Radiography, Thoracic/ or exp computer assisted tomography/ or positron emission tomography/ or multidetector computed tomography/ or exp nuclear magnetic resonance imaging/ or Thorax radiography/ or exp echography/ or computer assisted emission tomography/ or Endoscopy, Gastrointestinal/ or gastrointestinal endoscopy/ or ("computed tomography" or "computerized tomography" or "multidetector computerized tomography" or "magnetic resonance imaging" or "positron emission tomography" or (CT or PET or MRI or TRUS or TUS or ERUS or EUS or MD-CT or x-ray) or ((endorectal or endoscop$ or transrectal or transabdominal) and ultrasound) or imag$).mp
4	Combine	1 and 2 and 3
5	English	limit 4 to english language
6	Human	limit 5 to human
7	1980–2013	limit 6 to yr="1980 - 2013"
8	Humans	limit 7 to humans
9	Publication Types	8 not (letter/ or editorial/ or news/ or comment/ or case report.mp. or case reports/ or note/ or conference paper/ or (letter or editorial or news or comment or case reports or conference abstract$).pt.)
10	Publication Types	8 and case series
11	Combine	9 or 10
12	Dedupe	remove duplicates from 11

Table A-4. EMBASE/MEDLINE (presented in OVID syntax) – safety search

Set #	Concept	Search Statement
1	Imaging technology controlled vocabulary	exp Tomography, Emission-Computed/ae, mo or exp Tomography, X-Ray Computed/ae, mo or exp Magnetic Resonance Imaging/ae, mo or Endosonography/ae, mo or nuclear magnetic resonance imaging/ae or nuclear magnetic resonance imaging agent/ae, to or endoscopic echography/ae
2	Imaging technology keywords	("computed tomography" or "computerized tomography" or "magnetic resonance imaging" or "positron emission tomography" or (endoscop$ adj ultrasound)).ti,ab.
3	Imaging technology set	1 or 2
4	Radiation & contrast media controlled vocabulary	Radiation injury/ or Contrast Medium/ae or Radiation Injuries/ or Contrast Media/ae, to
5	Radiation & contrast media injuries related to imaging technologies	3 and 4
6	Imaging technologies and related harms	3 or 5
7	Harms & adverse events controlled vocabulary and keywords	Medical error/ or Medical errors/ or (harm or harms or (adverse adj2 (effect or effects or reaction or reactions or event or events or outcome or outcomes))).ti,ab.
8	Technologies and harms/adverse events	6 and 7
9	English	limit 8 to English language
10	Human	limit 9 to human
11	Date	limit 10 to yr=""2008 – 2013"
12	Humans	limit 11 to humans
13	Dedupe	remove duplicates from 12
14	Eliminate certain publication types	13 not (letter/ or editorial/ or news/ or comment/ or case report.mp. or case reports/ or note/ or conference paper/ or (letter or editorial or news or comment or case reports or conference abstract$).pt.)
15	Add in case series	13 and case series.mp.
16	Combine for final set	14 or 15

OVID Syntax:

$ or * = truncation character (wildcard)
ADJ*n* = search terms within a specified number (*n*) of words from each other in any order
/ = search as a subject heading (note that terms preceded by an asterisk are searched as a major subject headings)
exp = "explodes" controlled vocabulary term (e.g., expands search to all more specific related terms in the vocabulary's hierarchy)
.de. = limit controlled vocabulary heading
.fs. = floating subheading
.hw. = limit to heading word
.md. = type of methodology (PsycINFO)
.mp. = combined search fields (default if no fields are specified)
.pt. = publication type
.ti. = limit to title
.tw. = limit to title and abstract fields

Table A-5. PubMed

Set #	Concept	Search Statement
1	Subsets	(inprocess[sb] OR publisher[sb] OR pubmednotmedline[sb])
2	Colorectal cancer keywords	(Colon*[tiab] OR colorectal[tiab] OR rect*[tiab] OR rectal[tiab] OR rectum[tiab]) AND (cancer*[tiab] OR tumo*[tiab] OR tumor*[tiab] OR tumour*[tiab] OR neoplas*[tiab] OR carcinoma*[tiab] OR Adenocarcinoma[tiab])
3	Staging title keywords	(stag*[tiab] OR restag*[tiab] OR re-stag*[tiab])
4	Imaging technologies keywords	(("computerized tomography" OR "multidetector computerized tomography" OR "magnetic resonance imaging" OR "positron emission tomography") OR (intraoperative OR laparoscopic OR surgical) OR (CT OR PET OR MRI OR US OR ERUS OR EUS OR MD-CT OR x-ray) OR ((endorectal OR endoscopic OR laparoscopic OR transrectal OR transabdominal) and (ultrasound OR US)) OR imag* OR image OR imaging)
5	Combine	#1 AND #2 AND #3 AND #4

Table A-6. PubMed – safety search

Set #	Concept	Search Statement
1	Imaging technology	((computed tomography OR computerized tomography OR magnetic resonance imaging OR positron emission tomography OR (endoscop* AND ultrasound)))
2	Contrast/imaging agents	((imaging OR imag* OR contrast) AND (medium* OR agent*)
3	Radiation	((Radiation AND (image OR imaging OR imag* OR injury)))
4	Combine	#1 AND (#2 OR #3)
5	Safety	((medical error* OR harm* OR harm OR harms OR (adverse AND (effect OR effects OR reaction OR reactions OR event OR events OR outcome OR outcomes))))
6	Combine	(#1 OR #4) AND #5
7	Subsets	#6 AND (inprocess[sb] OR publisher[sb] OR pubmednotmedline[sb])
8	Date filter	Filters: published in the last 5 years

PubMed Syntax:

- * = truncation character (wildcard)
- [ti] = limit to title field
- [tiab] = limit to title and abstract fields
- [tw] = text word

Table A-7. Cochrane Library databases

Set #	Concept	Search Statement
1	Colorectal Cancer MeSH	MeSH descriptor: [Colorectal Neoplasms] explode all trees
2	Staging MeSH	MeSH descriptor: [Neoplasm Staging] explode all trees
3	Imaging Technologies MeSH	MeSH descriptor: [Diagnostic Imaging] explode all trees
4	Staging MeSH and keywords	#2 or (stag* or restag* or re-stag*):ti,ab,kw
5	Colorectal cancer MeSH and keywords	#1 or ((Colon or colorectal or rect*) and (cancer* or tumo* or neoplas* or carcinoma* or adenocarcinoma*)):ti,kw,ab
6	Imaging technologies MeSH and keywords	#3 or ("computed tomography" or "computerized tomography" or "multidetector computerized tomography" or "magnetic resonance imaging" or "positron emission tomography" or ultrasound or CT or PET or MRI or US or ERUS or EUS or MD-CT or MDCT or x-ray or imag*):ti,ab,kw
7	Combine	#4 and #5 and #6

Cochrane Library Syntax:

* = truncation character (wildcard)

The Cochrane Library via the Wiley platform is menu-driven.

Appendix B. Excluded Studies

Systematic Review Inclusion Criteria

Not a Systematic Review

Bipat S, Zwinderman AH, Bossuyt PM, et al. Multivariate random-effects approach: for meta-analysis of cancer staging studies. Acad Radiol. 2007 Aug;14(8):974-84

Dedemadi G, Wexner SD. Complete response after neoadjuvant therapy in rectal cancer: to operate or not to operate. Dig Dis. 2012;30 Suppl 2:109-17

Hartman RI, Chang CY, Wo JY, et al. Optimizing adjuvant treatment decisions for stage T2 rectal cancer based on mesorectal node size. A decision analysis. Acad Radiol. 2013 Jan;20(1):79-89

Heriot AG, Grundy A, Kumar D. Preoperative staging of rectal carcinoma. Br J Surg. 1999 Jan;86(1):17-28

Lejeune C, Bismuth MJ, Conroy T, et al. Use of a decision analysis model to assess the cost-effectiveness of 18F-FDG PET in the management of metachronous liver metastases of colorectal cancer. J Nucl Med. 2005 Dec;46(12):2020-8

Sautter-Bihl ML, Hohenberger W, Fietkau R, et al. MRI-based treatment of rectal cancer: is prognostication of the recurrence risk solid enough to render radiation redundant? Ann Surg Oncol. 2013 Sept 4. Epub ahead of Print.

Not High Quality

Leufkens AM, van den Bosch MA, van Leeuwen MS, et al. Diagnostic accuracy of computed tomography for colon cancer staging: a systematic review. Scand J Gastroenterol. 2011 Jul;46(7-8):887-94

Parnaby CN, Bailey W, Balasingam A, et al. Pulmonary staging in colorectal cancer: a review. Colorectal Dis. 2012 Jun;14(6):660-70

Puli SR, Bechtold ML, Reddy JB, et al. Can endoscopic ultrasound predict early rectal cancers that can be resected endoscopically? A meta-analysis and systematic review. Dig Dis Sci. 2010 May;55(5):1221-9

van der Parrdt MP, Zagers MB, Beets-Tan RGH, et al. Patients who undergo preoperative chemoradiotherapy for locally advanced rectal cancer restaging by using diagnostic MR imaging: a systematic review and meta-analysis. Radiology. 2013 Oct;269(1):101-12

Vriens D, de Geus-Oei LF, van der Graaf WT, et al. Tailoring therapy in colorectal cancer by PET-CT. Q J Nucl Med Mol Imaging. 2009 Apr;53(2):224-44

Patients Not Diagnosed With Cancer Before Enrollment

Brush J, Boyd K, Chappell F, et al. The value of FDG positron emission tomography/computerised tomography (PET/CT) in pre-operative staging of colorectal cancer: a systematic review and economic evaluation. Health Technol Assess. 2011 Sep;15(35):1-192, iii-iv

Not Reporting Staging Outcomes

Nordholm-Carstensen A, Wille-Jorgensen PA, Jorgensen LN, et al. Indeterminate pulmonary nodules at colorectal staging: a systematic review of predictive parameters for malignancy. Ann Surg Oncol. 2013 Nov;20(12):4022-30

Mixed Types of Cancer, Colorectal Not Reported Separately

Gao G, Gong B, and Shen W. Meta-analysis of the additional value of integrated ^{18}FDG PET-CT for tumor distant metastasis staging: comparison with ^{18}FDG PET alone and CT alone. Surg Oncol. 2013 Sept;22(3):195-200

Published Prior to 2009

Bipat S, Glas AS, Slors FJ, et al. Rectal cancer: local staging and assessment of lymph node involvement with endoluminal US, CT, and MR imaging--a meta-analysis. Radiology. 2004 Sep;232(3):773-83

Facey K, Bradbury I, Laking G, et al. Overview of the clinical effectiveness of positron emission tomography imaging in selected cancers. Health Technol Assess. 2007 Oct;11(44):iii-iv

Harewood GC. Assessment of publication bias in the reporting of EUS performance in staging rectal cancer. Am J Gastroenterol. 2005 Apr;100(4):808-16

Kwok H, Bissett IP, Hill GL. Preoperative staging of rectal cancer. Int J Colorectal Dis. 2000 Feb;15(1):9-20

Lahaye MJ, Engelen SM, Nelemans PJ, et al. Imaging for predicting the risk factors--the circumferential resection margin and nodal disease--of local recurrence in rectal cancer: a meta-analysis. Semin Ultrasound CT MR. 2005 Aug;26(4):259-68

Purkayastha S, Tekkis PP, Athanasiou T, et al. Diagnostic precision of magnetic resonance imaging for preoperative prediction of the circumferential margin involvement in patients with rectal cancer. Colorectal Dis. 2007 Jun;9(5):402-11

Skandarajah AR, Tjandra JJ. Preoperative loco-regional imaging in rectal cancer. ANZ J Surg. 2006 Jun;76(6):497-504

Tytherleigh MG, Warren BF, Mortensen NJ. Management of early rectal cancer. Br J Surg. 2008 Apr;95(4):409-23

Wiering B, Krabbe PF, Jager GJ, et al. The impact of Fluor-18-deoxyglucose-positron emission tomography in the management of colorectal liver metastases: a systematic review and metaanalysis. Cancer. 2005 Dec 15;104(12):2658-70

Primary Article Inclusion Criteria

All Patients Reported on Already in Pomerri et al. 2011[163]

Maretto I, Pomerri F, Pucciarelli S, et al. The potential of restaging in the prediction of pathologic response after preoperative chemoradiotherapy for rectal cancer. Ann Surg Oncol. 2007 Feb;14(2):455-61

Different Reference Standards for Different Groups of Patients

Squillaci E, Manenti G, Mancino S, et al. Staging of colon cancer: whole-body MRI vs. whole-body PET-CT--initial clinical experience. Abdom Imaging. 2008 Nov-Dec;33(6):676-88

Does Not Report on One of the Test Comparisons of Interest

Adi-Atmaka T. Transrectal ultrasonography; preoperative staging of rectal cancer. Croat J Gastroenterol Hepatol. 1992;1(1):35-9

Agrawal N, Fowler AL, Thomas MG. The routine use of intra-operative ultrasound in patients with colorectal cancer improves the detection of hepatic metastases. Colorectal Dis. 2006 Mar;8(3):192-4

Badger SA, Devlin PB, Neilly PJ, et al. Preoperative staging of rectal carcinoma by endorectal ultrasound: is there a learning curve? Int J Colorectal Dis. 2007 Oct;22(10):1261-8

Faneyte IF, Dresen RC, Edelbroek MA, et al. Pre-operative staging with positron emission tomography in patients with pelvic recurrence of rectal cancer. Dig Surg. 2008;25(3):202-7

Heneghan JP, Salem RR, Lange RC, et al. Transrectal sonography in staging rectal carcinoma: the role of gray-scale, color-flow, and Doppler imaging analysis. AJR Am J Roentgenol. 1997;169(5):1247-52

Huppertz A, Franiel T, Wagner M, et al. Whole-body MRI with assessment of hepatic and extraabdominal enhancement after administration of Gadoxetic acid for staging of rectal carcinoma. Acta Radiol. 2010

Oct;51(8):842-50

Itano S, Fuchimoto S, Hamada F, et al. The clinical significance of CT in the preoperative diagnosis of colon and rectal cancer. Hiroshima J Med Sci. 1986 Dec;35(4):309-15

Kalantzis Ch, Markoglou C, Gabriel P, et al. Endoscopic ultrasonography in the preoperative staging of colorectal cancer. Hepatogastroenterology. 2002 May-Jun;49(45):683-6

Petersen H, Nielsen MJ, Hoilund-Carlsen M, et al. PET/CT may change diagnosis and treatment in cancer patients. Dan Med Bull. 2010 Sep;57(9)

Ruers TJ, Wiering B, van der Sijp JR, et al. Improved selection of patients for hepatic surgery of colorectal liver metastases with (18)F-FDG PET: a randomized study. J Nucl Med. 2009 Jul;50(7):1036-41

Sabbagh C, Fuks D, Joly JP, et al. Is there a role for endoscopic ultrasonography in evaluation of the left liver in colorectal liver metastasis patients selected for right hepatectomy. Surg Endosc. 2009 Dec;23(12):2816-21

Spatz J, Holl G, Sciuk J, et al. Neoadjuvant chemotherapy affects staging of colorectal liver metastasis--a comparison of PET, CT and intraoperative ultrasound. Int J Colorectal Dis. 2011 Feb;26(2):165-71

Steele SR, Martin MJ, Place RJ. Flexible endorectal ultrasound for predicting pathologic stage of rectal cancers. Am J Surg. 2002 Aug;184(2):126-30

Tamandl D, Herberger B, Gruenberger B, et al. Adequate preoperative staging rarely leads to a change of intraoperative strategy in patients undergoing surgery for colorectal cancer liver metastases. Surgery. 2008 May;143(5):648-57

Tytherleigh MG, Ng VV, Pittathankal AA, et al. Preoperative staging of rectal cancer by magnetic resonance imaging remains an imprecise tool. ANZ J Surg. 2008 Mar;78(3):194-8

Zacherl J, Scheuba C, Imhof M, et al. Current value of intraoperative sonography during surgery for hepatic neoplasms. World J Surg. 2002 May;26(5):550-4

Does Not Report One of the Outcomes of Interest

Chun HK, Choi D, Kim MJ, et al. Preoperative staging of rectal cancer: comparison of 3-T high-field MRI and endorectal sonography. AJR Am J Roentgenol. 2006 Dec;187(6):1557-62

Phang PT, Gollub MJ, Loh BD, et al. Accuracy of endorectal ultrasound for measurement of the closest predicted radial mesorectal margin for rectal cancer. Dis Colon Rectum. 2012 Jan;55(1):59-64

Shinya S, Sasaki T, Nakagawa Y, et al. The efficacy of diffusion-weighted imaging for the detection of colorectal cancer. Hepatogastroenterology. 2009 Jan-Feb;56(89):128-32

Experimental Technology

Fuchsjager MH, Maier AG, Schima W, et al. Comparison of transrectal sonography and double-contrast MR imaging when staging rectal cancer. AJR Am J Roentgenol. 2003 Aug;181(2):421-7

Giovannini M, Bories E, Pesenti C, et al. Three-dimensional endorectal ultrasound using a new freehand software program: results in 35 patients with rectal cancer. Endoscopy. 2006 Apr;38(4):339-43

Haji A, Ryan S, Bjarnason I, et al. Colonoscopic high frequency mini-probe ultrasound is more accurate than conventional computed tomography in the local staging of colonic cancer. Colorectal Dis. 2012 Aug;14(8):953-9

Kam MH, Wong DC, Siu S, et al. Comparison of magnetic resonance imaging-Fluorodeoxyglucose positron emission tomography fusion with pathological staging in rectal cancer. Br J Surg. 2010 Feb;97(2):266-8

Lahaye MJ, Beets GL, Engelen SM, et al. Locally advanced rectal cancer: MR imaging for restaging after neoadjuvant radiation therapy with concomitant chemotherapy. Part II. What are the criteria to predict involved lymph nodes? Radiology. 2009 Jul;252(1):81-91

Maier AG, Kersting-Sommerhoff B, Reeders JW, et al. Staging of rectal cancer by double-contrast MR imaging using the rectally administered superparamagnetic iron oxide contrast agent Ferristene and IV gadodiamide injection: results of a multicenter phase II trial. J Magn Reson Imaging. 2000 Nov;12(5):651-60

Mezzi G, Arcidiacono PG, Carrara S, et al. Endoscopic ultrasound and magnetic resonance imaging for restaging rectal cancer after radiotherapy. World J Gastroenterol. 2009 Nov 28;15(44):5563-7

Veit-Haibach P, Kuehle CA, Beyer T, et al. Diagnostic accuracy of colorectal cancer staging with whole-body PET/CT colonography. JAMA. 2006 Dec 6;296(21):2590-600

Wallengren NO, Holtas S, Andren-Sandberg A, et al. Rectal carcinoma: double-contrast MR imaging for preoperative staging. Radiology. 2000 Apr;215(1):108-14

Wang X, Lv D, Song H, et al. Multimodal preoperative evaluation system in surgical decision making for rectal cancer: a randomized controlled trial. Int J Colorectal Dis. 2010 Mar;25(3):351-8

Fewer Than 10 Patients

Tio TL, Tytgat GN. Comparison of blind transrectal ultrasonography with endoscopic transrectal ultrasonography in assessing rectal and perirectal diseases. Scand J Gastroenterol Suppl. 1986;123:104-11

Mixed Group of Patient Types, Data Not Reported Separately by Group

Adeyemo D, Hutchinson R. Preoperative staging of rectal cancer: pelvic MRI plus abdomen and pelvic CT. Does extrahepatic abdomen imaging matter? A case for routine thoracic CT. Colorectal Dis. 2009 Mar;11(3):259-63

Blomqvist L, Machado M, Rubio C, et al. Rectal tumour staging: MR imaging using pelvic phased-array and endorectal coils vs endoscopic ultrasonography. Eur Radiol. 2000;10(4):653-60

Boutkan H, Luth W, Meyer S, et al. The impact of intraoperative ultrasonography of the liver on the surgical strategy of patients with gastrointestinal malignancies and hepatic metastases. Eur J Surg Oncol. 1992 Aug;18(4):342-6

Butch RJ, Stark DD, Wittenberg J, et al. Staging rectal cancer by MR and CT. AJR Am J Roentgenol. 1986 Jun;146(6):1155-60

Fernandez-Esparrach G, Ayuso-Colella JR, Sendino O, et al. EUS and magnetic resonance imaging in the staging of rectal cancer: a prospective and comparative study. Gastrointest Endosc. 2011 Aug;74(2):347-54

Georgakopoulos A, Pianou N, Kelekis N, et al. Impact of 18F-FDG PET/CT on therapeutic decisions in patients with colorectal cancer and liver metastases. Clin Imaging. 2013 May-June;37(3);536-41

Grassetto G, Fornasiero A, Bonciarelli G, et al. Additional value of FDG-PET/CT in management of "solitary" liver metastases: preliminary results of a prospective multicenter study. Mol Imaging Biol. 2010 Apr;12(2):139-44

Haijnen LA, Lambregts DMJ, Mondal D, et al. Diffusion-weighted MR imaging in primary rectal cancer staging demonstrates but does not characterize lymph nodes. Eur Radiol. 2013 July 3 Epub ahead of print.

Harnsberger JR, Charvat P, Longo WE, et al. The role of intrarectal ultrasound (IRUS) in staging of rectal cancer and detection of extrarectal pathology. Am Surg. 1994 Aug;60(8):571-6; discussion 576-7

Hunerbein M, Schlag PM. Three-dimensional endosonography for staging of rectal cancer. Ann Surg. 1997 Apr;225(4):432-8

Kim JC, Cho YK, Kim SY, et al. Comparative study of three-dimensional and conventional endorectal ultrasonography used in rectal cancer staging. Surg Endosc. 2002 Sep;16(9):1280-5

Kulinna C, Eibel R, Matzek W, et al. Staging of rectal cancer: diagnostic potential of multiplanar reconstructions with MDCT. AJR Am J Roentgenol. 2004 Aug;183(2):421-7

Manenti G, Ciccio C, Squillaci E, et al. Role of combined DWIBS/3D-CE-T1w whole-body MRI in tumor staging: comparison with PET-CT. Eur J Radiol. 2012 Aug;81(8):1917-25

Mathur P, Smith JJ, Ramsey C, et al. Comparison of CT and MRI in the pre-operative staging of rectal adenocarcinoma and prediction of circumferential resection margin involvement by MRI. Colorectal Dis. 2003 Sep;5(5):396-401

Mizukami Y, Ueda S, Mizumoto A, et al. Diffusion-weighted magnetic resonance imaging for detecting lymph node metastasis of rectal cancer. World J Surg. 2011 Apr;35(4):895-9

Rifkin MD, Ehrlich SM, Marks G. Staging of rectal carcinoma: prospective comparison of endorectal US and CT. Radiology. 1989 Feb;170(2):319-22

Sinha R, Verma R, Rajesh A, et al. Diagnostic value of multidetector row CT in rectal cancer staging: comparison of multiplanar and axial images with histopathology. Clin Radiol. 2006 Nov;61(11):924-31

Swartling T, Kalebo P, Derwinger K, et al. Stage and size using magnetic resonance imaging and endosonography in neoadjuvantly-treated rectal cancer. World J Gastroenterol. 2013 June;19(21):3263-71

Thomson V, Pialat JB, Gay F, et al. Whole-body MRI for metastases screening: a preliminary study using 3D VIBE sequences with automatic subtraction between noncontrast and contrast enhanced images. Am J Clin Oncol. 2008 Jun;31(3):285-92

More Than 50 Percent of Patients Lost

Barbaro B, Valentini V, Manfredi R. Combined modality staging of high risk rectal cancer. Rays. 1995 Apr-Jun;20(2):165-81

Caseiro-Alves F, Goncalo M, Cruz L, et al. Water enema computed tomography (WE-CT) in the local staging of low colorectal neoplasms: comparison with transrectal ultrasound. Abdom Imaging. 1998 Jul-Aug;23(4):370-4

Cho YB, Chun HK, Kim MJ, et al. Accuracy of MRI and 18F-FDG PET/CT for restaging after preoperative concurrent chemoradiotherapy for rectal cancer. World J Surg. 2009 Dec;33(12):2688-94

Holdsworth PJ, Johnston D, Chalmers AG, et al. Endoluminal ultrasound and computed tomography in the staging of rectal cancer. Br J Surg. 1988 Oct;75(10):1019-22

Panzironi G, De Vargas Macciucca M, et al. Preoperative locoregional staging of rectal carcinoma: comparison of MR, TRUS and Multislice CT. Personal experience. Radiol Med. 2004 Apr;107(4):344-55

Shami VM, Parmar KS, Waxman I. Clinical impact of endoscopic ultrasound and endoscopic ultrasound-guided fine-needle aspiration in the management of rectal carcinoma. Dis Colon Rectum. 2004 Jan;47(1):59-65

No Reference Standard

Aljebreen AM, Azzam NA, Alzubaidi AM, et al. The accuracy of multi-detector row computerized tomography in staging rectal cancer compared to endoscopic ultrasound. Saudi J Gastroenterol. 2013 May;19(3):108-12

Cipe G, Ergul N, Hasbahceci M, et al. Routine use of positron-emission tomography/computed tomography for staging of primary colorectal cancer: does it affect clinical management? World J Surg Oncol. 2013 Feb;11(1):49-56

Maizlin ZV, Brown JA, So G, et al. Can CT replace MRI in preoperative assessment of the circumferential resection margin in rectal cancer? Dis Colon Rectum. 2010 Mar;53(3):308-14

Vliegen R, Dresen R, Beets G, et al. The accuracy of Multi-detector row CT for the assessment of tumor invasion of the mesorectal fascia in primary rectal cancer. Abdom Imaging. 2008 Sep-Oct;33(5):604-10

Not a Clinical Study

MRI better than FDG-PET at detecting liver tumors. Oncology (Huntingt). 2005 Aug;19(9):1176

Beets-Tan RG, Beets GL, Van De Velde CJ. Staging in colorectal cancer. Eur J Cancer Suppl. 2005 Oct;3(3):361-6

Fasih N, Virmani V, Walsh C, et al. Double-contrast magnetic resonance imaging in preoperative evaluation of rectal cancer: use of aqueous jelly as luminal contrast. Can Assoc Radiol J. 2011 May;62(2):122-4

Garcia-Aguilar J. Transanal endoscopic microsurgery following neoadjuvant chemoradiation therapy in rectal cancer: a word of caution about patient selection? Dis Colon Rectum. 2013 Jan;56(1):1-3

Hamm B. Multi-detector CT of the abdomen. Eur Radiol. 2003;13

Husband JE, Sharma B. Radiological staging of gastrointestinal and breast tumours. Br J Surg. 2006 May;93(5):513-5

Iyer R. Imaging colorectal cancer. Semin Roentgenol. 2006 Apr;41(2):113-20

Low RN. MRI of colorectal cancer. Abdom Imaging. 2002 Jul-Aug;27(4):418-24

McCarthy S. Proper staging and monitoring of colonic carcinoma. Postgrad Radiol. 1986;6(3):195-201

Moadel RM, Feng J, Freeman LM. PET/CT in the evaluation of colorectal carcinoma. Appl Radiol. 2008 Nov;37(11):33-42

Moss AA. Imaging of colorectal carcinoma. Radiology. 1989 Feb;170(2):308-10

Rembacken BJ, Cairns A, Kudo S, et al. Images of early rectal cancer. Endoscopy. 2004 Mar;36(3):223-33

Romanini A, Cellini N, Coco C. Combined diagnostic techniques for clinical staging of cancer of the rectum. Rays. 1982;7(1):39-51

Wiggers T. Staging of rectal cancer. Br J Surg. 2003 Aug;90(8):895-6

Wong WD. Transrectal ultrasound: accurate staging for rectal cancer. J Gastrointest Surg. 2000 Jul-Aug;4(4):338-9

Not Colorectal Cancer

Kim JC, Kim HC, Yu CS, et al. Efficacy of 3-dimensional endorectal ultrasonography compared with conventional ultrasonography and computed tomography in preoperative rectal cancer staging. Am J Surg. 2006 Jul;192(1):89-97

Koch J, Halvorsen RA Jr, Levenson SD, et al. Prospective comparison of catheter-based endoscopic sonography versus standard endoscopic sonography: evaluation of gastrointestinal-wall abnormalities and staging of gastrointestinal malignancies. J Clin Ultrasound. 2001 Mar-Apr;29(3):117-24

Lai DT, Fulham M, Stephen MS, et al. The role of whole-body positron emission tomography with [18F]fluorodeoxyglucose in identifying operable colorectal cancer metastases to the liver. Arch Surg. 1996 Jul;131(7):703-7

Miyake KK, Nakamoto Y, Togashi K. Dual-time-point 18F-FDG PET/CT in patients with colorectal cancer: clinical value of early delayed scanning. Ann Nucl Med. 2012 Jul;26(6):492-500

Suzuki C, Torkzad MR, Tanaka S, et al. The importance of rectal cancer MRI protocols on interpretation accuracy. World J Surg Oncol. 2008 Aug 20;6:89

Yamashita S, Masui T, Katayama M, et al. T2-weighted MRI of rectosigmoid carcinoma: comparison of respiratory-triggered fast spin-echo, breathhold fast-recovery fast spin-echo, and breathhold single-shot fast spin-echo sequences. J Magn Reson Imaging. 2007 Mar;25(3):511-6

Not in English

Balena V, Martino D, Lorusso F, et al. Endorectal ultrasound and magnetic resonance imaging (MRI) scan in rectal cancer: a comparative study. Arch Ital Urol Androl. 2010 Dec;82(4):259-61

Bianchi P, Ceriani C, Palmisano A, et al. A prospective comparison of endorectal ultrasound and pelvic magnetic resonance in the preoperative staging of rectal cancer. Ann Ital Chir. 2006 Jan-Feb;77(1):41-6

Dinter DJ, Hofheinz RD, Hartel M, et al. Preoperative staging of rectal tumors: comparison of endorectal ultrasound, hydro-CT, and high-resolution endorectal MRI. Onkologie. 2008 May;31(5):230-5

Feifel G. Does endorectal sonography influence treatment of rectal cancer? Z Gastroenterol. 1989;27:102-7

Palko A, Gyulai C, Fedinecz N, et al. Water enema CT examination of rectum cancer by reduced amount of water. ROFO Fortschr Geb Rontgenstr Nuklearmed. 2000 Nov;172(11):901-4

Rifkin MD, Marks G. Endorectal sonography in prospective staging of rectal cancer. Z Gastroenterol. 1989;27(Spec

Iss):98-101

Siegel R, Dresel S, Koswig S, et al. Response to preoperative short-course radiotherapy in locally advanced rectal cancer: Value of 18F-Fluorodeoxyglucose positron emission tomography. Onkologie. 2008;31(4):166-72

Obsolete Technology

Cellini N, Coco C, Maresca G, et al. Clinical staging of rectal cancer: a study on 126 patients. Rays. 1986 Jan-Apr;11(1):69-79

Gearhart SL, Frassica D, Rosen R, et al. Improved staging with pretreatment positron emission tomography/computed tomography in low rectal cancer. Ann Surg Oncol. 2006 Mar;13(3):397-404

Kwak JY, Kim JS, Kim HJ, et al. Diagnostic value of FDG-PET/CT for lymph node metastasis of colorectal cancer. World J Surg. 2012 Aug;36(8):1898-905

Pegios W, Vogl J, Mack MG, et al. MRI diagnosis and staging of rectal carcinoma. Abdom Imaging. 1996 May-Jun;21(3):211-8

Reed WP, Haney PJ, Elias EG. Ethiodized oil emulsion enhanced computerized tomography in the preoperative assessment of metastases to the liver from the colon and rectum. Surg Gynecol Obstet. 1986;162(2):131-6

Ruhlmann J, Schomburg A, Bender H, et al. Fluorodeoxyglucose whole-body positron emission tomography in colorectal cancer patients studied in routine daily practice. Dis Colon Rectum. 1997 Oct;40(10):1195-204

Yu SL, Tsang YM, Liang PC, et al. Application of magnetic resonance images in gastrointestinal malignancies. Chin J Radiol. 2003 Oct;28(5):269-75

Zagoria RJ, Schlarb CA, Ott DJ, et al. Assessment of rectal tumor infiltration utilizing endorectal MR imaging and comparison with endoscopic rectal sonography. J Surg Oncol. 1997 Apr;64(4):312-7

Zerhouni EA, Rutter C, Hamilton SR, et al. CT and MR imaging in the staging of colorectal carcinoma: report of the Radiology Diagnostic Oncology Group II. Radiology. 1996 Aug;200(2):443-51

Off Topic

Baumann T, Ludwig U, Pache G, et al. Continuously moving table MRI with sliding multislice for rectal cancer staging: image quality and lesion detection. Eur J Radiol. 2010 Mar;73(3):579-87

Fischer MA, Nanz D, Hany T, et al. Diagnostic accuracy of whole-body MRI/DWI image fusion for detection of malignant tumours: a comparison with PET/CT. Eur Radiol. 2011 Feb;21(2):246-55

Ippolito D, Monguzzi L, Guerra L, et al. Response to neoadjuvant therapy in locally advanced rectal cancer: assessment with diffusion-weighted MR imaging and 18FDG PET/CT. Abdom Imaging. 2012 Dec;37(6):1032-40

Izadpanah A, Hosseini SV, Jalli R, et al. Efficacy of endorectal ultrasonography in preoperative staging of rectal carcinoma. Saudi Med J. 2005 Aug;26(8):1308-10

Killeen T, Banerjee S, Vijay V, et al. Magnetic resonance (MR) pelvimetry as a predictor of difficulty in laparoscopic operations for rectal cancer. Surg Endosc. 2010 Dec;24(12):2974-9

Kim SH, Lee JM, Hong SH, et al. Locally advanced rectal cancer: added value of diffusion-weighted MR imaging in the evaluation of tumor response to neoadjuvant chemo- and radiation therapy. Radiology. 2009 Oct;253(1):116-25

Lambregts DM, Vandecaveye V, Barbaro B, et al. Diffusion-weighted MRI for selection of complete responders after chemoradiation for locally advanced rectal cancer: a multicenter study. Ann Surg Oncol. 2011 Aug;18(8):2224-31

Patients Not Diagnosed With Cancer Before Enrollment

Arulampalam T, Costa D, Visvikis D, et al. The impact of FDG-PET on the management algorithm for recurrent colorectal cancer. Eur J Nucl Med. 2001 Dec;28(12):1758-65

Dirisamer A, Halpern BS, Flory D, et al. Performance of integrated FDG-PET/contrast-enhanced CT in the staging and restaging of colorectal cancer: comparison with PET and enhanced CT. Eur J Radiol. 2010 Feb;73(2):324-8

Kim CK, Kim SH, Choi D, et al. Comparison between 3-T magnetic resonance imaging and multi-detector row computed tomography for the preoperative evaluation of rectal cancer. J Comput Assist Tomogr. 2007 Nov-Dec;31(6):853-9

Rollven E, Holm T, Glimelius B, et al. Potentials of high resolution magnetic resonance imaging versus computed tomography for preoperative local staging of colon cancer. Acta Radiol. 2013 Aug;54(7):722-30

Soyka JD, Veit-Haibach P, Strobel K, et al. Staging pathways in recurrent colorectal carcinoma: is contrast-enhanced 18F-FDG PET/CT the diagnostic tool of choice? J Nucl Med. 2008 Mar;49(3):354-61

Sudakoff GS, Gasparaitis A, Michelassi F, et al. Endorectal color Doppler imaging of primary and recurrent rectal wall tumors: preliminary experience. AJR Am J Roentgenol. 1996 Jan;166(1):55-61

Retrospective Study That Did Not Enroll All or Consecutive Patients

Beer-Gabel M, Assouline Y, Zmora O, et al. A new rectal ultrasonographic method for the staging of rectal cancer. Dis Colon Rectum. 2009 Aug;52(8):1475-80

Maas M, Lambregts DM, Lahaye MJ, et al. T-staging of rectal cancer: accuracy of 3.0 Tesla MRI compared with 1.5 Tesla. Abdom Imaging. 2012 Jun;37(3):475-81

Tateishi U, Maeda T, Morimoto T, et al. Non-enhanced CT versus contrast-enhanced CT in integrated PET/CT studies for nodal staging of rectal cancer. Eur J Nucl Med Mol Imaging. 2007 Oct;34(10):1627-34

Appendix C. Evidence Tables

Systematic Reviews

Table C-1. Included systematic reviews: design

Study	Modalities Studied	Staging	Condition	Databases Searched	Dates Searched	Inclusion Criteria	Primary Method of Analysis	Funding	Statement of No Conflicts Given
Gall et al. 2013[84]	ERUS (mini-probe)	Pre-operative staging	Colorectal cancer	MEDLINE, EMBASE, Cochrane	Through January 2013	Studies of mini-probe ERUS for staging of colon cancer or mixed colorectal that used histopathology as the reference standard and staged using the TNM system	Bivariate and hierarchical summary receiver operating characteristics model	National Institute of Health Research Biomedical Research Center	Yes
Lu et al. 2012[87]	PET/CT, PET	Pre-operative staging	Colorectal cancer	MEDLINE, PubMed, EMBASE	Through February 2 012	Full-length published articles of nodal staging by PET or PET/CT in patients with colorectal cancer with sufficient data reported to derive 2x2 tables	Random-effects or fixed-effects pooling of sensitivity/specificity separately	China Medical University Hospital, Taiwan Department of Health grants	Yes

Table C-1. Included systematic reviews: design (continued)

Study	Modalities Studied	Staging	Condition	Databases Searched	Dates Searched	Inclusion Criteria	Primary Method of Analysis	Funding	Statement of No Conflicts Given
Al-Sukhni et al. 2012[86]	MRI	Pre-operative staging	Rectal cancer	MEDLINE, EMBASE, Cochrane	January 2000 to March 2011	English-language original published reports of MRI using a phase-array coil, histopathology as the reference standard, and sufficient data reported to construct 2x2 tables	Bivariate random-effects model and hierarchical summary receiver operating characteristics model	Grant from Cancer Services Innovation Partnership	No
van Kessel et al. 2012[198]	MRI, CT, PET/CT	Interim re-staging	Colorectal cancer	MEDLINE and EMBASE	Through May 2011	Full-length published articles of patients diagnosed with unresectable colorectal liver metastases who were treated with neoadjuvant chemotherapy and then re-staged by imaging.	Random-effects or fixed-effects pooling of sensitivities	No external funding	Yes

Table C-1. Included systematic reviews: design (continued)

Study	Modalities Studied	Staging	Condition	Databases Searched	Dates Searched	Inclusion Criteria	Primary Method of Analysis	Funding	Statement of No Conflicts Given
Niekel et al. 2010[15]	PET/CT, CT	Pre-operative staging	Colorectal liver metastases	MEDLINE, EMBASE, Cochrane, CINAHL, Web of Science	January 1990 to January 20 10	Prospective full-length published articles with at least 10 patients with histopathologically proven colorectal cancer undergoing evaluation for liver metastases that reported sufficient data to allow calculation of sensitivity and specificity	Random-effects or fixed-effects pooling of sensitivity/specificity separately	None reported	Yes
Dighe et al. 2010[16]	CT	Pre-operative staging, N and T	Colon cancer primarily, a few studies mixed colorectal	MEDLINE, EMBASE, Cochrane	Through March 5, 2009	Published preoperative N staging using histopathology as the reference standard and sufficient data reported to calculate TP, TN, FP, and FN	Bivariate random-effects model	NIHR Biomedical Research Centre (Royal Marsden Hospital)	No
Puli et al. 2009[85]	Endoscopic US	Pre-operative staging	Rectal cancer	MEDLINE, PubMed, EMBASE, CINAHL, Cochrane, DARE, Healthstar	1966 to January 2008	Full-length published studies of rectal cancer N staging confirmed by surgical histology that reported sufficient data to construct 2x2 tables	Random-effects or fixed-effects pooling of sensitivity/specificity separately	Not funded	Yes

Table C-1. Included systematic reviews: design (continued)

Study	Modalities Studied	Staging	Condition	Databases Searched	Dates Searched	Inclusion Criteria	Primary Method of Analysis	Funding	Statement of No Conflicts Given
Puli et al. 2009[14]	Endoscopic US	Pre-operative staging	Rectal cancer	MEDLINE, PubMed, EMBASE, CINAHL, Cochrane, DARE, Healthstar	1980 to January 2008	Full-length published studies of T staging rectal cancer with endoscopic ultrasound using surgical histology as the reference standard and sufficient data to construct 2x2 tables	Random-effects or fixed-effects pooling of sensitivity/specificity separately	not funded	Yes

CT=Computed tomography; DARE=Database of Abstracts of Reviews of Effects; FN=false-negative; FP=false-positive; MRI=Magnetic resonance imaging; PET/CT=positron emission tomography/computed tomography; PET=positron emission tomography; TN=true negative; TP=true positive; US=ultrasound

Table C-2. Included systematic reviews: results

Study	Number of Articles	Number of Patients	Study Quality	Reference Standard	Publication Bias	Primary Results	Author's Conclusion
Gall et al. 2013[84]	10 ERUS total; 5 colon only, 5 mixed colorectal	642 total; 210 colon only.	All studies had 8 or more of the 14 QUADAS items; 60% had 10 of the 14 items.	Histopathology	Not assessed	T1: sensitivity 91%, specificity 98%; T2: sensitivity 78%, specificity 94%; T3/T4: sensitivity 97%, specificity 90%; N: sensitivity 63%, specificity 82%.	Mini-probe ERUS is effective in staging colorectal cancer.
Lu et al. 2012[87]	8 PET, 2 PET/CT	83 PET/CT, 326 PET	On the Cochrane Diagnostic Tests tool, the mean quality score was 59.2%, Range: 33% to 83%	Histopathology	Not assessed	The sensitivity of PET for detecting involved lymph nodes was 42.9% (95% CI, 36.0% to 50.0%), the specificity was 87.9% (95% CI, 82.6% to 92.0%)	There is no solid evidence to support the routine clinical application of PET (PET/CT) in the pretherapeutic evaluation of lymph node status in patients with colorectal cancer.

Table C-2. Included systematic reviews: results (continued)

Study	Number of Articles	Number of Patients	Study Quality	Reference Standard	Publication Bias	Primary Results	Author's Conclusion
Al-Sukhni et al. 2012[86]	19 studies for T stage, 12 studies for N stage, 10 studies for CRM	1,986 patients for T stage, 1,249 patients for N stage, 986 patients for CRM	62% of the studies had 10 or more of the 13 modified QUADAS items	Histopathology	Not assessed	MRI for N: sensitivity 77% (95% CI, 69% to 84%), specificity 71% (95% CI, 59% to 81%). MRI for T: sensitivity 87% (95% CI, 81% to 92%), specificity 75% (95% CI, 68% to 80%). MRI for CRM: sensitivity 77% (95% CI, 57% to 90%), specificity 94% [95% CI, 8% to 97%]	MRI has good accuracy for both CRM and T category and should be considered for preoperative rectal cancer staging. In contrast, lymph node assessment is poor on MRI.
van Kessel et al. 2012[198]	5 studies of CT, 3 studies of MRI, 2 studies of PET/CT (some studies evaluated more than one modality)	221 CT, 54 MRI, 137 PET/CT	QUADAS was used to exclude 7 studies prior to data extraction	Intraoperative ultrasound, histopathology of resected lesions, and patient followup (8.8% were confirmed only by patient followup)	Funnel plots did not show any evidence of gross publication bias	There was heterogeneity in the sensitivity of MRI and PET/CT but not for CT. CT sensitivity: 54.5% (95% CI 46.7 to 62.1%) MRI sensitivity: 69.9% (95% CI 65.6 to 73.9%) PET/CT sensitivity: 51.7% (95% CI 37.8 to 65.4%)	MRI appears to be the most appropriate imaging modality for interim restaging of colorectal cancer liver metastases. If MRI is unavailable, CT should be used. PET/CT is strongly affected by neoadjuvant chemotherapy.

Table C-2. Included systematic reviews: results (continued)

Study	Number of Articles	Number of Patients	Study Quality	Reference Standard	Publication Bias	Primary Results	Author's Conclusion
Niekel et al. 2010[15]	25 CT, 18 MRI, 5 PET/CT	Total 3,391	65% of the studies had 6 or more of the 10 modified QUADAS items	A mixture of histopathology and clinical followup	There was no evidence of publication bias on funnel plots	Sensitivity of CT for liver mets: 83.6% Sensitivity of MRI for liver mets: 88.2% Sensitivity of PET/CT for liver mets: data were too limited	MRI imaging is the preferred first-line modality for evaluating colorectal liver metastases in patients who have not previously undergone therapy.
Dighe et al. 2010[16]	19 total; 17 reported on T stage, 15 on N stage	907 total, 784 T stage, 674 N stage	53% of studies scored 12 or higher on the QUADAS items	Histopathology	There was some evidence of publication bias, with smaller studies reporting a higher diagnostic odds ratio for nodal detection	CT T1/T2 differentiate from T3/T4 sensitivity 86% (95% CI, 78 to 92%), specificity 78% (95% CI, 71 to 84%) CT T3 from T4 sensitivity 92% (95% CI, 87 to 95%), specificity 81% (70 to 89%) CT N stage sensitivity 70% (95% CI, 59 to 80%), specificity 78% (95% CI, 66 to 0.86%)	Preoperative staging CT accurately distinguishes between tumors confined to the bowel wall and those invading beyond the MP; however, it is significantly poorer at identifying nodal status. MDCT provides the best results

Table C-2. Included systematic reviews: results (continued)

Study	Number of Articles	Number of Patients	Study Quality	Reference Standard	Publication Bias	Primary Results	Author's Conclusion
Puli et al. 2009[85]	35	2,732	All of the studies fulfilled 4 to 5 out of the 14 QUADAS items	Histopathology	There was no evidence of publication bias on funnel plots	ERUS for N staging: sensitivity of 73.2% (95% CI, 70.6 to 75.6); specificity 75.8% (95% CI, 73.5 to 78.0) likelihood ratios + 2.84 (95% CI, 2.16 to 3.72), -0.42 (95% CI, 0.33 to 0.52)	ERUS is an important and accurate diagnostic tool for evaluating nodal metastasis of rectal cancers. This meta-analysis shows that the sensitivity and specificity of ERUS is moderate.

Table C-2. Included systematic reviews: results (continued)

Study	Number of Articles	Number of Patients	Study Quality	Reference Standard	Publication Bias	Primary Results	Author's Conclusion
Puli et al. 2009[14]	42	5,039	All of the studies fulfilled 4 to 5 out of the 14 QUADAS items	Histopathology	There was no evidence of publication bias on funnel plots	ERUS for T1: sensitivity 87.8% (95% CI, 85.3 to 90.0), specificity 98.3% (95% CI; 97.8 to 98.7), +LR 44.0 (22.7 to 85.5), -LR 0.16 (0.13 to 0.23) ERUS for T2: sensitivity 80.5% (77.9 to 82.9), specificity 95.6 (94.9 to 96.3), +LR 17.3 (11.9 to 24.9), -LR 0.22 (0.17 to 0.29) ERUS for T3: sensitivity 96.4% (95.4 to 97.2), specificity 90.6 (89.5 to 91.7), +LR 8.9 (6.8 to 11.8), -LR 0.06 (0.04 to 0.09) ERUS for T4: sensitivity 95.4 (92.4 to 97.5), specificity 98.3 (97.8 to 98.7), +LR 37.6 (19.9 to 71.0), -LR 0.14 (0.09 to 0.23)	As a result of the demonstrated sensitivity and specificity, ERUS should be the investigation of choice to T stage rectal cancers. The sensitivity of ERUS is higher for advanced disease than for early disease, ERUS should be strongly considered for T staging of rectal cancers.

95% CI=95% confidence interval; CRM=circumferential resection margin; CT=confidence interval; ERUS=endorectal ultrasound; MDCT=multiphase detector computed tomography; MRI=magnetic resonance imaging; N stage=nodal stage; PET=positron emission tomography; PET/CT=positron emission tomography/computed tomography; QUADAS=quality assessment tool for diagnostic accuracy studies; T stage=tumor stage

Table C-3. Included systematic reviews: quality assessment

Study	Does the review mention that a protocol was published prior to conduct of the systematic review?	Was a comprehensive search strategy performed and reported?	Was the search strategy appropriate to address the Key Questions of this CER?	Was a list of included and excluded studies provided?	Was the application of inclusion/exclusion criteria unbiased and consistent?	Are the inclusion/exclusion criteria appropriate to address the Key Questions of this CER?	Was there duplicate study selection and data extraction?	Were the included studies described?	Was the individual study quality assessed?	Was the method of study quality assessment consistent with that recommended by the Methods Guide?	Was the quality of the individual studies used appropriately in formulating conclusions?	Were the methods used to combine the findings of the studies appropriate?	Was the likelihood of publication bias assessed?	Have the authors reported sources of funding and/or disclosed conflicts of interest?
Gall et al. 2013[84]	No	Yes	Yes	Yes	Yes	Yes	No	No	Yes	Yes	No	Yes	No	Yes
Lu et al. 2012[87]	No	Yes	Yes	Yes	Yes	Yes	Yes	Yes	Yes	Yes	Yes	Yes	No	Yes
Al-Sukhni et al. 2010[86]	No	Yes	Yes	Yes	Yes	Yes	Yes	Yes	Yes	Yes	Yes	Yes	No	Yes
van Kessel et al. 2012[198]	No	Yes	Yes	Yes	Yes	Yes	No	Yes	Yes	Yes	Yes	Yes	Yes	Yes
Dighe et al. 2010[16]	No	Yes	Yes	Yes	Yes	Yes	No	Yes	Yes	Yes	No	Yes	Yes	Yes
Niekel et al. 2010[15]	Yes	Yes	Yes	Yes	Yes	Yes	Yes	Yes	Yes	Yes	Yes	Yes	Yes	Yes
Puli et al. 2009[85]	No	Yes	Yes	Yes	Yes	Yes	Yes	No	Yes	Yes	No	Yes	Yes	Yes
Puli et al. 2009[14]	No	Yes	Yes	Yes	Yes	Yes	Yes	Yes	Yes	Yes	No	Yes	Yes	Yes

CER=Comparative effectiveness review.

CT Versus ERUS

Table C-4. Study design: CT versus ERUS

Study	Outcomes Reported	Design	Prospective?	Funded by	Setting	Country
Wickramasinghe and Samarasekera 2012[126]	Changes in management–rectal staging	One group (cohort or case series)	Prospective	Not reported	University	Sri Lanka
Ju et al. 2009[99]	Preoperative rectal T and N staging accuracy	One group (cohort or case series)	Unclear	Not reported	University	China
Huh et al. 2008[164]	Interim rectal restaging accuracy; factors affecting accuracy	One group (cohort or case series)	Retrospective	Not reported	University	Korea
Harewood et al. 2002[127]	Changes in management–rectal staging	One group (cohort or case series)	Prospective	Not reported	Mayo clinic	USA
Kim et al. 1999[100]	Preoperative rectal and T and N staging accuracy	One group (cohort or case series)	Unclear	Not reported	University	Korea
Osti et al. 1997[101]	Preoperative rectal T and N staging accuracy	One group (cohort or case series)	Unclear	Not reported	University	Italy
Ramana et al. 1997[102]	Preoperative rectal and T and N staging accuracy	One group (cohort or case series)	Prospective	Not reported	Medical College	India
Fleshman et al. 1992[116]	Preoperative rectal staging with intervening radiation therapy	One group (cohort or case series)	Prospective	Not reported	University	USA
Milsom et al. 1992[118]	Recurrent rectal staging accuracy	One group (cohort or case series)	Prospective	Not reported	Community based private nonprofit clinic	USA
Goldman et al. 1991[103]	Preoperative rectal and T and N staging accuracy	One group (cohort or case series)	Prospective	Not reported	Community hospital	Sweden

Table C-4. Study design: CT versus ERUS (continued)

Study	Outcomes Reported	Design	Prospective?	Funded by	Setting	Country
Pappalardo et al. 1990[104]	Preoperative rectal T and N staging accuracy	One group (cohort or case series)	Prospective	Not reported	University	Italy
Rotte et al. 1989[105]	Preoperative rectal T and N staging accuracy	One group (cohort or case series)	Unclear	Not reported	Cancer institute	Germany
Waizer et al. 1989[106]	Preoperative rectal T staging accuracy	One group (cohort or case series)	Prospective	Not reported	Community hospital	Israel
Beynon et al. 1986[107]	Preoperative rectal T staging accuracy	One group (cohort or case series)	Prospective	Cancer Research Campaign	Teaching hospital	United Kingdom
Kramann and Hildebrandt 1986[108]	Preoperative rectal T staging accuracy	One group (cohort or case series)	Unclear	Not reported	University	Germany
Rifkin and Wechsler 1986[109]	Preoperative rectal T and N staging accuracy	One group (cohort or case series)	Prospective	Not reported	University	USA
Rifkin and Marks 1986[110]	Preoperative rectal and T and N staging accuracy	One group (cohort or case series)	Prospective	Not reported	University	USA
Romano et al. 1985[111]	Preoperative rectal T staging accuracy	One group (cohort or case series)	Unclear	Not reported	Medical school	Italy

USA=United States of America.

Table C-5. Patient details: CT versus ERUS

Study	Type of Cancer	Age	% Male
Wickramasinghe and Samarasekera 2012[126]	Primary rectal	Mean: 57.3 (Range: 23–80)	50%
Ju et al. 2009[99]	Primary rectal	Mean: 61 (Range: 32–78)	53.8%
Huh et al. 2008[164]	Locally advanced rectal, within 7 cm from the anal verge	Mean: 54.0 (Range: 31–80)	62.7%
Harewood et al. 2002[127]	Primary rectal	Mean: 65.3 (SD: 3.2)	57%
Kim et al. 1999[100]	Primary rectal	Not reported	Not reported
Osti et al. 199[101]	Primary rectal	Mean: 61 (Range: 36–74)	54.0%
Ramana et al. 1997[102]	Rectal carcinoma	35–70	70%
Fleshman et al. 1992[116]	Advanced rectal tumors	Not reported	57.8%
Milsom et al. 1992[118]	Recurrent rectal cancer	Median: 59 (Range: 31–68)	35%
Goldman et al. 1991[103]	Rectal cancer within 10 cm of the anal verge	Not reported	68.8%
Pappalardo et al. 1990[104]	Primary rectal	Not reported	57%
Rotte et al. 1989[105]	Primary rectal	Not reported	Not reported
Waizer et al. 1989[106]	Primary rectal within 10 cm of the anal verge	Mean: 65 (Range: 28–82)	Not reported
Beynon et al. 1986[107]	Primary rectal	Median: 67 (Range: 46–83)	Not reported
Kramann and Hildebrandt 1986[108]	Primary rectal	Mean: 61	62%
Rifkin and Wechsler 1986[109]	Primary rectal	Not reported	Not reported
Rifkin and Marks 1986[110]	Primary rectal	36–77	Not reported
Romano et al. 1985[111]	Primary rectal, located in the lower 2/3s of the rectum	Not reported	Not reported

cm=Centimeter; CT=Computed tomography; ERUS=endorectal ultrasonography SD=standard deviation.

Table C-6. Imaging details: CT versus ERUS

Study	CT Contrast Agents	Type of CT	Bowel Prep for CT	Type of ERUS	MHz of ERUS	Bowel Prep for ERUS
Wickramasinghe and Samarasekera 2012[126]	None reported	10 mm spiral	Enema	360 degree Olympus GFUM 20 endoanal probe	10	None reported
Ju et al. 2009[99]	Air in the rectum	5 mm slices	None reported	Not reported	8 and 10	Enema
Huh et al. 2008[164]	Rectal contrast material	5 to 7 mm slices	None reported	Rubber sheath, 360 rotating	7.5 or 10	None reported
Harewood et al. 2002[127]	Oral and IV	10 mm slices	None reported	Radial scanning	7.5 and 12	None reported
Kim et al. 1999[100]	Rectal contrast material	5 mm slices	None reported	Rotating transducer	7.5	Enema
Osti et al. 1997[101]	Oral gastrografin, rectal air inflation, with and without IV nonionic contrast agent	10 mm slices	None reported	Not reported	7	None reported
Ramana et al. 1997[102]	Oral urograffin and IV urograffin	10 mm slices	None reported	20 mm rigid inserted to 10 mm depth	5.0 and 7.5	None reported
Fleshman et al. 1992[116]	Oral	Not reported	None reported	360 rotating probe, at least 16 cm long	7.5	None reported
Milsom et al. 1992[118]	IV and intraluminal contrast	6 mm transaxial; heavy patients had 9 mm	None reported	Not reported	7.0 or 10.0	None reported
Goldman et al. 1991[103]	Oral contrast gastrografin; 4 patients had IV Omnipaque	9 mm slices	None reported	Transversely oriented radial scan plane	7	None reported
Pappalardo et al. 1990[104]	None reported	8 mm slices	None reported	Radial probe	Not reported	Enema
Rotte et al. 1989[105]	Oral contrast; 2 had rectal air	Not reported	None reported	Linear array scanner, 10 cm or 15 cm	3,5 or 7.0	None reported
Waizer et al. 1989[106]	None reported	Not reported	None reported	Rotating	4	None reported

C-14

Table C-6. Imaging details: CT versus ERUS, (continued)

Study	CT Contrast Agents	Type of CT	Bowel Prep for CT	Type of ERUS	MHz of ERUS	Bowel Prep for ERUS
Beynon et al. 1986[107]	Rectal and IV, type not mentioned	4 mm slices	None reported	Rotating endoprobe	Either 5.5 or 7.0	None reported
Kramann and Hildebrandt 1986[108]	3 patients had water in the rectum; the rest had air. 7 patients had IV iodinated contrast media	10 mm slices	None reported	Not reported	Not reported	None reported
Rifkin and Wechsler 1986[109]	None reported	Not reported	None reported	Radial and linear, at least 25 cm long	Not reported	None reported
Rifkin and Marks 1986[110]	None reported	10 mm slices	None reported	Not reported	4, 7, or 7.5	None reported
Romano et al. 1985[111]	Oral Gastrografin, and IV not named	10 mm spiral	Enema	12 cm long	3.5 for most patients, 7.5 for some	None reported

cm=Centimeter; CT=Computed tomography; ERUS=endorectal ultrasonography; IV=intravenous; mm=millimeter; MHz=megahertz.

Table C-7. Reported data: CT versus ERUS for preoperative primary rectal staging T

Study, N patients, Author's Conclusion	Outcomes	CT Reported T Stage Data	ERUS Reported T Stage Data	T stage by Pathology	CT T1	CT T2	CT T3	CT T4	ERUS T1	ERUS T2	ERUS T3	ERUS T4
Ju et al. 2009[99] 78 patients	Accuracy	70.5%	84.6%	pT1	0	7	0	0	7	0	0	0
	T1/T2 vs. T3/T4 Sensitivity	84.8%	93.4%	pT2	0	16	9	0	2	21	2	0
Conclusion: **ERUS is better**	T1/T2 vs. T3/T4 Specificity	71.9%	93.8%	pT3	0	7	22	4	0	2	27	2
				pT4	0	0	3	10	0	0	2	11
Kim et al. 1999[100] 89 patients had ERUS, of these 69 also had CT	Accuracy	65.2%	81.1%	pT1	NR	NR	NR	NR	NR	NR	NR	NR
	Overstaging	12/69 (17.4%)	9/89 (10.0%)	pT2	NR	NR	NR	NR	NR	NR	NR	NR
	Understaging	12/69 (17.4%)	8/89 (8.9%)	pT3	NR	NR	NR	NR	NR	NR	NR	NR
Conclusion: **ERUS is better**				pT4	NR	NR	NR	NR	NR	NR	NR	NR
Ramana et al. 1997[102] 10 patients	Accuracy	10%	90%	pT1	NR	NR	NR	NR	4	0	0	0
	T1/T2 vs. T3/T4 Sensitivity	Not reported	100%	pT2	NR	NR	NR	NR	0	1	0	0
Conclusion: **ERUS is better for early disease; CT is better for advanced disease**	T1/T2 vs. T3/T4 Specificity	Not reported	100%	pT3	NR	NR	NR	NR	0	0	4	0
				pT4	NR	NR	NR	1	0	0	1	0

Table C-7. Reported data: CT versus ERUS for preoperative primary rectal staging T (continued)

Study, N patients, Author's Conclusion	Outcomes	CT Reported T Stage Data	ERUS Reported T Stage Data	T stage by Pathology	CT T1	CT T2	CT T3	CT T4	ERUS T1	ERUS T2	ERUS T3	ERUS T4
Osti et al. 1997[101] 63 patients	Accuracy	74%	83%	pT1	0	3	0	0			0	0
	T1/T2 vs. T3/T4 Sensitivity	83%	91%	pT2	0	0	11	0			7	0
Conclusion: ERUS is better	T1/T2 vs. T3/T4 Specificity	62%	67%	pT3	0	0	4	0			32	0
				pT4	0	0	0	5			0	6
Goldman et al. 1991[103] 29 patients	Accuracy	52%	81%	pT1	NR	NR	NR	NR	NR	NR	NR	NR
	T1/T2 vs. T3/T4 Sensitivity	67%	90%	pT2	NR	NR	NR	NR	NR	NR	NR	NR
Conclusion: ERUS is better	T1/T2 vs. T3/T4 Specificity	27%	67%	pT3	NR	NR	NR	NR	NR	NR	NR	NR
	Overstaging Understaging	8/29 (27.6%) 6/29 (20.7%)	4/29 (13.8%) 2/29 (6.9%)	pT4	NR	NR	NR	NR	NR	NR	NR	NR
Pappalardo et al. 1990[104] 14 patients	Accuracy	77.8%	100%	pT1	1	0	0	0	1	0	0	0
	T1/T2 vs. T3/T4 Sensitivity	77.8%	100%	pT2	0	4	0	0	0	4	0	0
Conclusion: ERUS is better	T1/T2 vs. T3/T4 Specificity	100%	100%	pT3	0	2	6	0	0	0	7	0
				pT4	0	0	0	1	0	0	1	1
Rotte et al. 1989[105] 25 patients	Accuracy	76%	84%	pT1	0	0	0	0	0	0	0	0
	T1/T2 vs. T3/T4 Sensitivity	84.6%	81.3%	pT2	0	9	3	0	0	8	1	0
Conclusion:	T1/T2 vs.	75.0%	88.9%	pT3	0	2	9	1	0	3	11	0

Table C-7. Reported data: CT versus ERUS for preoperative primary rectal staging T (continued)

Study, N patients, Author's Conclusion	Outcomes	CT Reported T Stage Data	ERUS Reported T Stage Data	T stage by Pathology	CT T1	CT T2	CT T3	CT T4	ERUS T1	ERUS T2	ERUS T3	ERUS T4
ERUS is better	T3/T4 Specificity			pT4	0	0	0	1	0	0	0	2
Waizer et al. 1989[106] 58 had CT, of these 42 also had ERUS	Accuracy	65.5%	76.8%	pT1	NR	NR	NR	NR	NR	NR	NR	NR
	T1/T2 vs. T3/T4 Sensitivity	82.6%	88.8%	pT2	NR	NR	NR	NR	NR	NR	NR	NR
	T1/T2 vs. T3/T4 Specificity	NR	NR	pT3	NR	NR	NR	NR	NR	NR	NR	NR
				pT4	NR	NR	NR	NR	NR	NR	NR	NR
Conclusion: **ERUS is better**												
Beynon et al. 1986[107] 44 patients	Accuracy	82%	91%	pT1	NR	NR	NR	NR	NR	NR	NR	NR
	T1/T2 vs. T3/T4 Sensitivity	86%	94%	pT2	NR	NR	NR	NR	NR	NR	NR	NR
Conclusion: **ERUS is better**	T1/T2 vs. T3/T4 Specificity	62%	87%	pT3	NR	NR	NR	NR	NR	NR	NR	NR
	Overstaging Understaging	3/44 (6.8%) 5/44 (11.4%)	2/44 (4.5%) 2/44 (4.5%)	pT4	NR	NR	NR	NR	NR	NR	NR	NR
Kramann and Hildebrandt 1986[108] 29 patients	Accuracy	75.9%	93.1%	pT1	0	0	0	0	0	0	0	0
	T1/T2 vs. T3/T4 Sensitivity	95.0%	100.0%	pT2	0	4	5	0	0	7	2	0
	T1/T2 vs. T3/T4 Specificity	44.4%	77.8%	pT3	0	1	17	1	0	0	19	0
Conclusion: **ERUS is better**				pT4	0	0	0	1	0	0	0	1
Rifkin and Weschler. 1986[110a] 79 had ERUS,	Accuracy	69.0%	86.1%	pT1	NR	NR	NR	NR	NR	NR	NR	NR
	T1/T2 vs. T3/T4 Sensitivity	55%	83%	pT2	NR	NR	NR	NR	NR	NR	NR	NR

Table C-7. Reported data: CT versus ERUS for preoperative primary rectal staging T (continued)

Study, N patients, Author's Conclusion	Outcomes	CT Reported T Stage Data	ERUS Reported T Stage Data	T stage by Pathology	CT T1	CT T2	CT T3	CT T4	ERUS T1	ERUS T2	ERUS T3	ERUS T4
and 71 of these also had CT	T1/T2 vs. T3/T4 Specificity	79%	84%	pT3	NR	NR	NR	NR	NR	NR	NR	NR
				pT4	NR	NR	NR	NR	NR	NR	NR	NR
Conclusion: **ERUS is better**												
Rifkin et al. 1986[110a]	Accuracy	69%	93%	pT1	NR	NR	NR	NR	NR	NR	NR	NR
54 had ERUS, and 51 of these also had CT	T1/T2 vs. T3/T4 Sensitivity	55%	89%	pT2	NR	NR	NR	NR	NR	NR	NR	NR
	T1/T2 vs. T3/T4 Specificity	81%	86%	pT3	NR	NR	NR	NR	NR	NR	NR	NR
Conclusion: **ERUS is better**				pT4	NR	NR	NR	NR	NR	NR	NR	NR

C-19

Table C-7. Reported data: CT versus ERUS for preoperative primary rectal staging T (continued)

Study, N patients, Author's Conclusion	Outcomes	CT Reported T Stage Data	ERUS Reported T Stage Data	T stage by Pathology	CT T1	CT T2	CT T3	CT T4	ERUS T1	ERUS T2	ERUS T3	ERUS T4
Romano et al. 1985[111] 23 patients	Accuracy	82.6%	87.0%	pT1	NR	NR	NR	NR	NR	NR	NR	NR
	Overstaging	2/23 (8.7%)	1/23 (4.4%)	pT2	NR	NR	NR	NR	NR	NR	NR	NR
	Understaging	2/23 (8.7%)	2/23 (8.7%)	pT3	NR	NR	NR	NR	NR	NR	NR	NR
Conclusion: ERUS is better				pT4	NR	NR	NR	NR	NR	NR	NR	NR

[a] It is possible that these two studies are reporting on an overlapping patient population.

CT=Computed tomography; ERUS=endorectal ultrasound; NR=not reported; pT=pathologic tumor stage; T=tumor stage.

Table C-8. Reported data: CT versus ERUS for rectal staging N

Study, N patients, Author's Conclusion	Outcome	CT Reported N Stage Data	ERUS Reported N Stage Data	N stage by Pathology	CT N0	CT N1+2	ERUS N0	ERUS N1+2
Ju et al. 2009[99] 78 patients	Accuracy	61.5%	64.1%					
	N0 vs. N1/2 Sensitivity Specificity	60.6% 62.2%	54.5% 71.1%	pN0 pN1+2	28 13	17 20	32 15	13 18
Conclusion: **Neither was satisfactory**								
Kim et al. 1999[100] 89 patients had ERUS, of these 69 also had CT	Accuracy	63.5%	56.5%					
	N0 vs. N1/2 Sensitivity Specificity	56.0% 56.8%	53.3% 75.0%	pN0 pN1+2	25 11	19 14	30 10	21 24
Conclusion: **Neither was satisfactory**								
Ramana et al. 1997[102] 10 patients	Accuracy	60.0%	90.0%					
	N0 vs. N1/2 Sensitivity Specificity	33.3% 100%	83.3% 100%	pN0 pN1+2	4 4	0 2	4 1	0 5
Conclusion: **Neither was satisfactory**								
Osti et a. 1997[101] 63 patients	Accuracy	57%	66%					
	N0 vs. N1/2 Sensitivity Specificity	56% 57%	68% 64%	pN0 pN1+2	16 11	12 14	18 8	10 17
Conclusion: **Neither was satisfactory**								
Goldman et al. 1991[103] 29 patients	Accuracy	64%	68%					
	N0 vs. N1/2 Sensitivity Specificity	67% 62%	50% 88%	pN0 pN1+2	NR NR	NR NR	NR NR	NR NR
Conclusion: **Neither was satisfactory**								

Table C-8. Reported data: CT versus ERUS for rectal staging N

Study, N patients, Author's Conclusion	Outcome	CT Reported N Stage Data	ERUS Reported N Stage Data	N stage by Pathology	CT N0	CT N1+2	ERUS N0	ERUS N1+2
Pappalardo et al. 1990[104] 14 patients Conclusion: **ERUS is better**	Accuracy N0 vs. N1/2 Sensitivity Specificity	57.1% 37.5% 83.3%	85.7% 87.5% 83.3%	pN0 pN1+2	5 5	1 3	5 1	1 7
Rotte et al. 1989[105] 25 patients Conclusion: **Neither could be used for N staging**	Accuracy N0 vs. N1/2 Sensitivity Specificity	92.0% 33.3% 100%	92.0% 33.3% 100%	pN0 pN1+2	22 2	0 1	22 2	0 1
Rifkin and Weschler. 1986[110a] 79 had ERUS, and 71 of these also had CT Conclusion: **ERUS was slightly better**	Accuracy N0 vs. N1/2 Sensitivity Specificity	77.2% 23% 100%	88.6% 67% 91%	pN0 pN1+2	58 10	0 3	60 5	6 10
Rifkin et al. 1986[110a] 54 had ERUS, and 51 of these also had CT Conclusion: **ERUS is better**	Accuracy N0 vs. N1/2 Sensitivity Specificity	84.3% 20% 100%	83.3% 72% 86%	pN0 pN1+2	41 8	0 2	37 3	6 8

[a] It is possible that these two studies are reporting on an overlapping patient population.

CT=Computed tomography; ERUS=endorectal ultrasound; N=nodal stage; NR=not reported; pN=pathologic nodal stage.

Table C-9. Reported data: CT versus ERUS for rectal staging with intervening radiation therapy

Study	Type of Cancer, Number of Patients	Reference Standard	Reported T Stage Data	Reported N Stage Data	Which one was chosen as better by the study authors?
Fleshman et al. 1992[116]	Primary rectal treated with radiation, 19	Histopathology	CT had an overall accuracy of 53% vs. ERUS with an overall accuracy of 32%	The negative predictive value of both CT and ERUS was 100%	Preoperative radiation therapy makes both CT and ERUS less effective for local staging, but N node staging is very accurate

CT=Computed tomography; ERUS=endorectal ultrasound; N=nodal stage; T=tumor stage.

Table C-10. Reported data: CT versus ERUS for preoperative primary rectal staging changes in management

Study	Type of Cancer, Number of Patients	Design	Results	Conclusions
Wickramasinghe and Samarasekera et al. 2012[126]	Primary rectal, 24	All patients underwent ERUS and CT, and a treatment plan was created based on each assessment	Out of the 24 patients, 13 had a different stage assigned by the two different modalities. Of these, the treatment plan based on CT was changed in 6 patients after adding the ERUS information. The T stage was changed in 9 patients, and of these 5 had a change in management; the N stage changed in 5 patients, and of these only 1 had a change in management.	ERUS and CT have only a fair to moderate agreement for staging and deciding treatment. However, ERUS has a significant influence when deciding treatment protocols.
Harewood et al. 2002[127]	Primary rectal, 80	5 surgeons made treatment decisions on the basis of clinical data plus CT staging data; then they were given ERUS data, and changes in management were recorded	In 25 of 80 of patients (31%), adding the ERUS information prompted the surgeon to change the based-on-CT only treatment plan. In all cases of a change, the change was from proceeding directly to surgery to undergoing neoadjuvant therapy first instead. The study did not measure whether the change in management resulted in better patient outcomes.	Preoperative staging with CT plus ERUS resulted in more frequent use of preoperative neoadjuvant therapy than staging with CT alone.

CT=Computed tomography; ERUS=endorectal ultrasound; N=nodal stage; T=tumor stage.

Table C-11. Reported data: CT versus ERUS for preoperative recurrent rectal staging

Study	Type of Cancer, Number of Patients	Reference Standard	Reported T Stage Data	Reported N Stage Data	Reported M Stage	Which one was chosen as better by the study authors?
Milsom et al. 1992[118]	Recurrent rectal, 14	Histopathology	CT accurately predicted the extent of organ involvement in 8 patients vs. ERUS accurately predicted the extent of organ involvement in 11	Not reported	Not reported	ERUS was better than CT for assessing the extent of local recurrence

CT=Computed tomography; ERUS=endorectal ultrasound; M=metastases stage; N=nodal stage; T=tumor stage.

Table C-12. Reported data: CT versus ERUS for preoperative interim rectal restaging

Study	Type of Cancer, Number of Patients	Reference Standard	Reported T Stage Data	Reported N Stage Data	Reported M Stage	Which one was chosen as better by the study authors?
Huh et al. 2008[164]	Locally advanced rectal cancer, post radiochemotherapy, 83; 60 had ERUS and 80 had CT	Histopathology	For predicting the depth of invasion, CT overstaged 28 and understaged 15, for a total accuracy of 46.3% vs. ERUS that overstaged 22 and understaged 15 for a total accuracy of 38.3%.	For prediction of nodal involvement, CT had a sensitivity of 56.0% and a specificity of 74.5% vs. ERUS that had a sensitivity of 50.0% and a specificity of 81.1%	Not reported	Neither was selected as a good modality for restaging rectal cancer after neoadjuvant treatment

CT=Computed tomography; ERUS=endorectal ultrasound; M=metastases stage; N=nodal stage; T=tumor stage.

Table C-13. Reported data: factors affecting CT versus ERUS for preoperative interim rectal restaging

Study	Type of Cancer, Number of Patients	Reference Standard	Reported T Stage Data Factors	Reported N Stage Data Factors	Reported M Stage Factors
Huh et al. 2008[164]	Locally advanced rectal cancer, post radiochemotherapy, 83; 60 had ERUS and 80 had CT	Histopathology	Distance from anal verge- ERUS was much more accurate for ≤4 cm; ERUS was more accurate for T2 and T3 tumors than for T0, T1, or T4 tumors.	Time interval between treatment and surgery- ERUS was much more accurate for a longer (>7 weeks) interval; ERUS was more accurate for N0 than for N1 or N2	Not reported

CT=Computed tomography; ERUS=endorectal ultrasound; M=metastases stage; N=nodal stage; T=tumor stage.

MRI Versus ERUS

Table C-14. Study design: MRI versus ERUS

Study	Outcomes Reported	Design	Prospective?	Funded by	Setting	Country
Yimei et al. 2012[93]	Preoperative rectal T and N staging accuracy and changes in management for rectal staging	Two groups (controlled comparative)	Retrospective	Science and Technology Commission of Shanghai Municipality	University	China
Halefoglu et al. 2008[94]	Preoperative rectal T and N staging accuracy	One group (cohort or case series)	Unclear	Not reported	Training and research hospital	Turkey
Rafaelsen et al. 2008[188]	Factors affecting accuracy	One group (cohort or case series)	Retrospective	Not reported	Community hospital	Denmark
Bianchi et al. 2005[95]	Preoperative rectal T and N staging accuracy	One group (cohort or case series)	Unclear	Not reported	University	Italy
Brown et al. 2004[125]	Changes in management–rectal staging	One group (cohort or case series)	Prospective	Wales Office of Research and Development for Health and Social Care	University	United Kingdom
Starck et al. 1995[96]	Preoperative rectal T and N staging accuracy	One group (cohort or case series)	Prospective	Not reported	University	Sweden
Thaler et al. 1994[97]	Preoperative rectal T and N staging accuracy	One group (cohort or case series)	Prospective	Not reported	Community hospital	Italy
Waizer et al. 1991[98]	Preoperative rectal T staging accuracy	One group (cohort or case series)	Prospective	Not reported	Community hospital	Israel

Table C-15. Patient details: MRI versus ERUS

Study	Type of Cancer	Age	% Male
Yimei et al. 2012[93]	Primary rectal	Mean: 62 years (Range: 24–88)	59.7%
Halefoglu et al. 2008[94]	Primary rectal	Mean: 58.7 years (Range: 29–75)	44.1%
Rafaelsen et al. 2008[188]	Primary rectal	Mean: 69.1 years (Range: 38–89)	Not reported
Bianchi et al. 2005[95]	Resectable rectal cancer	Mean: 64 years (Range: 30–85)	Not reported
Brown et al. 2004[125]	Primary rectal	Range: 28–89	73.5%
Starck et al. 1995[96]	Primary rectal	Mean: 68 years (Range: 47–84)	68%
Thaler et al. 1994[97]	Primary rectal	Mean: 68.9 years (Range: 52–86)	67.8%
Waizer et al. 1991[98]	Primary rectal	Mean: 66 years (Range: 60–80)	33.3%

Table C-16. Imaging details: MRI versus ERUS

Study	Contrast Agents for MRI	Type of MRI	Bowel Prep for MRI	Type of ERUS	MHz of ERUS	Bowel Prep for ERUS
Yimei et al. 2012[93]	None reported	3T magnet, weighting not reported	None reported	360-degree radial echo-endoscope	Not reported	None reported
Halefoglu et al. 2008[94]	None reported	1.5T magnet, T2 weighted, pelvic phased-array coil	None used	Superficial endoprobe	7 and 10	Enema
Rafaelsen et al. 2008[188]	None used	1.5T magnet, T2 weighted, pelvic coil	No, but was done on the same day had an enema for US	Forward-looking	7.5 MHz; harmonic, color, power, 3D	Enema
Bianchi et al. 2005[95]	Air in rectum	1.0T magnet, T1 and T2 weighting, body coil	Enema	Flexible	7.5	No
Brown et al. 2004[125]	Not reported	Magnet not reported, T2 weighted	Not reported	Radial scanning	7.5 and 10	Yes
Starck et al. 1995[96]	None used	0.3T magnet, T1 and T2 weighting	No	1846 Bruel and Kjar (no details)	7	None reported
Thaler et al. 1994[97]	Not reported	0.5T magnet, T1 and T2 weighting	Cleansing with polyethylene glycol	Combison rotating	5, 7.5, 10	Enema
Waizer et al. 1991[98]	Not reported	0.5T magnet, T1 and T2 weighting	Enema	Real time rotating	7	None reported

Table C-17a. Reported data: MRI versus ERUS for rectal staging T

Study N Patients, Author's Conclusion	Outcome	MRI Reported T Stage Data	ERUS Reported T Stage Data	T Stage by Pathology	MRI T1	MRI T2	MRI T3	MRI T4	ERUS T1	ERUS T2	ERUS T3	ERUS T4
Yimei et al. 2012[93] 69 MRI, 60 ERUS	Accuracy	79.7%	83.3%	pT1	6	0	0	0	14	1	0	0
	T1/T2 vs. T3/T4 Sensitivity	92.9%	89.7%	pT2	6	12	3	0	1	14	1	0
	T1/T2 vs. T3/T4 Specificity	88.9%	96.8%	pT3	0	3	21	1	0	2	11	3
				pT4	0	0	1	16	1	0	1	11
Conclusion: ERUS is better for early-stage, but MRI is better for locally advanced												
Halefoglu et al. 2008[94] 34 patients	Accuracy	89.70%	85.29%	pT1	1	0	0	0	0	1	0	0
	T1/T2 vs. T3/T4 Sensitivity	95.8%	87.5%	pT2	0	5	4	0	0	4	5	0
	T1/T2 vs. T3/T4 Specificity	60.0%	50.0%	pT3	0	1	18	2	0	3	18	0
				pT4	0	0	0	3	0	0	1	2
Conclusion: MRI was slightly superior to ERUS												

Table C-17a. Reported data: MRI versus ERUS for rectal staging T (continued)

Study N Patients, Author's Conclusion	Outcome	MRI Reported T Stage Data	ERUS Reported T Stage Data	T Stage by Pathology	MRI T1	MRI T2	MRI T3	MRI T4	ERUS T1	ERUS T2	ERUS T3	ERUS T4
Starck et al. 1995[96] 35 had MRI, but tumor not detected in 3) 34 of these also had ERUS Conclusion: **ERUS is better; MRI seems to underestimate the extension of rectal tumors**	Accuracy	66%	88%	pT1	0	0	0	0	1	1	0	0
	T1/T2 vs. T3/T4 Sensitivity	78.3%	91.3%	pT2	4	5	0	0	0	8	1	0
	T1/T2 vs. T3/T4 Specificity	100.0%	90.9%	pT3	1	4	18	0	0	2	21	0
				pT4	0	0	0	0	0	0	0	0

Table C-17a. Reported data: MRI versus ERUS for rectal staging T (continued)

Study N Patients, Author's Conclusion	Outcome	MRI Reported T Stage Data	ERUS Reported T Stage Data	T Stage by Pathology	MRI T1	MRI T2	MRI T3	MRI T4	ERUS T1	ERUS T2	ERUS T3	ERUS T4
Thaler et al. 1994[97] 34 patients	Accuracy	82.3%	88.2%	pT1	NR	NR	NR	NR	NR	NR	NR	NR
	T1/T2 vs. T3/T4 Sensitivity	76.9%	92.3%	pT2	NR	NR	NR	NR	NR	NR	NR	NR
Conclusion: ERUS is better, except when there is stenosis	T1/T2 vs. T3/T4 Specificity	85.7%	85.7%	pT3	NR	NR	NR	NR	NR	NR	NR	NR
				pT4	NR	NR	NR	NR	NR	NR	NR	NR
Waizer et al. 1991[98] 13 patients	Accuracy	76.9%	84.6%	pT1	0	0	0	0	1	0	0	0
	T1/T2 vs. T3/T4 Sensitivity	88.9%	88.9%	pT2	0	3	1	0	0	2	1	0
Conclusion: Both have a place in staging	T1/T2 vs. T3/T4 Specificity	75.0%	75.0%	pT3	0	1	7	1	0	1	8	0
				pT4	0	0	0	0	0	0	0	0

CI=Confidence interval; ERUS=endorectal ultrasound; MRI=magnetic resonance imaging; NR=not reported; pT=pathologic tumor stage; T=tumor stage.

Table C-17b. Reported data: MRI versus ERUS for rectal staging T

Study N Patients, Author's Conclusion		MRI Reported T Stage Data	ERUS Reported T Stage Data	Modality	Overstaged	Understaged
Bianchi et al. 2005[95]	Accuracy	BC: 43% (95% CI, 0.39 to 0.75) PC: 71% (95% CI, 0.52 to 0.91)	70% (95% CI, 0.65 to 0.90)	ERUS	0.17	0.12
49 ERUS; of these, 28 BC MRI, 21 PC MRI	T1/T2 vs. T3/T4 Sensitivity	Not reported	Not reported	MRI BC	0.25	0.32
	T1/T2 vs. T3/T4 Specificity	Not reported	Not reported	MRI PC	0.14	0.14
Conclusion: MRI using a phased-array coil was the single best method						

BC=Body coil; PC=multi-channel phased-array 4 coil system.

Table C-18a. Reported data: MRI versus ERUS for rectal staging N

Study, N Patients, Author's Conclusion	Outcomes	MRI Reported N Stage Data	ERUS Reported N Stage Data	Stage by Pathology	MRI Stage	ERUS versus Pathological Stage
Yimei et al. 2012[93] 69 MRI, 60 ERUS	Accuracy	76.8%	70.0%	pN0	N0: 31 N1+2: 4	N0: 31 N1+2: 9
	N0 vs. N1/2 Sensitivity	64.7%	55.0%	pN1+2	N0: 12 N1+2: 22	N0: 9 N1+2: 11
Conclusion: **ERUS is better for early stage, but MRI is better for locally advanced**	N0 vs. N1/2 Specificity	88.6%	77.5%			
Halefoglu et al. 2008[228] 34 patients	Accuracy	74.50%	76.47%	pN0	N0: 8 N1: 11 N2:0	N0:7 N1: 12 N2: 0
	N0 vs. N1/2 Sensitivity	61.76%	52.94%	pN1	N0:1 N1: 8 N2: 0	N0: 2 N1: 7 N2: 0
Conclusion: **MRI is as good as ERUS**	N0 vs. N1/2 Specificity	80.88%	84.31%	pN2	N0: 1 N1: 0 N2: 5	N0: 2 N1: 0 N2:4
Starck et al. 1995[96] 35 MRI; 34 of these also had ERUS	Accuracy	72%	71%	pN0	N0: 14 N1+2: 4	N0: 13 N1+2: 4
	N0 vs. N1/2 Sensitivity	64.3%	64.3%	pN1+2	N0: 5 N1+2: 9	N0: 5 N1+2: 9
Conclusion: **Neither was reliable for N stage**	N0 vs. N1/2 Specificity	77.8%	76.5%			
Thaler et al. 1994[97] 25 patients	Accuracy	60.0%	80.0%	pN0	N0: 10 N1+2: 1	N0: 11 N1+2: 0
	N0 vs. N1/2 Sensitivity	35.7%	64.3%	pN1+2	N0: 9 N1+2: 5	N0: 5 N1+2: 9
Conclusion: **Neither was reliable for N stage**	N0 vs. N1/2 Specificity	90.9%	100.0%			

CI=Confidence interval; ERUS=endorectal ultrasound; MRI=magnetic resonance imaging; N=nodal stage; pN=pathologic nodal stage; pT=pathologic tumor stage; T=tumor stage.

Table C-18b. Reported data: MRI versus ERUS for rectal staging N

Study, N Patients, Author's Conclusion	Outcomes	MRI Reported N Stage Data	ERUS Reported N Stage Data
Bianchi et al. 2005[95] 49 ERUS; of these, 28 BC MRI, 21 PC MRI	Accuracy	BC: 64% (95% CI, 47 to 82) PC: 76% (95% CI, 58 to 94)	63% (95% CI, 50 to 80)
	N0 vs. N1/2 Sensitivity	BC: 62% PC: 63%	47%
Conclusion: **No method was satisfactory, but MRI using phased-array coils was marginally better**	N0 vs. N1/2 Specificity	BC: 80% PC: 80%	80%
	Overstaging	BC: 0.14 PC: 0.21	0.10
	Understaging	BC: 0.21 PC: 0.14	0.27

BC=Body coil; PC=Multi-channel phased-array 4 coil system.

Table C-19. Reported data: MRI versus ERUS for preoperative primary rectal staging changes in management

Study	Type of Cancer, Number of Patients	Design	Results	Conclusions
Yimei et al. 2012[93]	Rectal cancer, 69 had MRI, 60 had ERUS	For each patient, 3 treatment strategies were designed: S-1 was based solely on MRI or ERUS staging; S-2 was based on MRI or ERUS staging plus any other clinical information available and was the actual treatment performed; S-3 was based on the pathological results after surgery (the reference strategy).	Compared with the reference strategy, MRI based strategy would have undertreated 3/69 cases and overtreated 11/69, with accurate treatment of 55/69, vs. ERUS based strategy would have undertreated 4/60 and overtreated 10/60 with accurate treatment of 46/60. The actual treatment (S-2) using MRI plus clinical would have undertreated 2/69 and overtreated 2/69 vs. ERUS plus clinical would have undertreated 2/60 and overtreated 2/60.	The actual treatment accuracy using MRI plus clinical information was 94.2% vs. 91.7% for ERUS plus clinical information; the treatment accuracy using MRI alone was 76.7% vs. 66.7% for ERUS.
Brown et al. 2004[125]	Rectal cancer, 98	Treatment strategies were devised based on MRI or ERUS staging; the patients were then treated using all available information; and histopathology was used to define the "correct" treatment that should have been used.	Compared with the reference strategy, MRI based strategy would have undertreated 11/98 and overtreated 1/98 patients with accurate treatment of 86/98, vs. ERUS based strategy would have undertreated 32/98 and overtreated 19/98 with accurate treatment of 47/98. The majority of errors with ERUS were understaging locally advanced (T4) cancers as T3 and overstaging T1/T2 as T3.	The treatment accuracy using MRI was 87.8% vs. 48.0% for ERUS

ERUS=Endorectal ultrasonography; MRI=magnetic resonance imaging.

Table C-20. Reported data: factors affecting MRI versus ERUS for preoperative rectal staging

Study	Type of Cancer, Number of Patients	Reference Standard	Reported T Stage Data Factors	Reported N Stage Data Factors	Author's Conclusions
Rafaelsen et al. 2008[188]	Rectal cancer, 134; experienced radiologist examined 58 ERUS/ 75 MRI and inexperienced radiologist examined 76 ERUS/59 MRI	Histopathology	For predicting penetration of the rectal wall by ERUS, experienced reader had a sensitivity of 93% and specificity of 83%, accuracy 90%; inexperienced reader had a sensitivity of 75% and specificity of 46%, accuracy 66%; by MRI, experienced reader had a sensitivity of 96% and a specificity of 74%, accuracy 88%; inexperienced reader had a sensitivity of 77%, specificity 40%, accuracy 68%.	For predicting involvement of lymph nodes by ERUS, experienced reader had a sensitivity of 45%, specificity 79%, accuracy of 67%; inexperienced reader had a sensitivity of 23%, specificity of 77%, accuracy 66%; by MRI, experienced reader had a sensitivity of 77%, specificity of 64%, accuracy 68%; inexperienced reader had a sensitivity of 50%, specificity 67%, accuracy 61%.	Reader experience had a statistically significant effect on the accuracy of preoperative prediction of tumor involvement of the rectal wall.

ERUS=Endorectal ultrasonography; MRI=magnetic resonance imaging.

MRI Versus PET/CT

Table C-21. Study design: MRI versus PET/CT

Study	Outcomes Reported	Design	Prospective?	Funded by?	Setting	Country
Kim et al. 2011[88]	Preoperative rectal N staging	One group (cohort or case series)	Retrospective	Yonsei University College of Medicine	University	South Korea

Table C-22. Patient details: MRI versus PET/CT

Study	Type of Cancer	Age	% Male
Kim et al. 2011[88]	Primary rectal	Mean: 62 years (Range: 46–83)	70%

Table C-23. Imaging details: MRI versus PET/CT

Study	Contrast Agents for MRI	Type of MRI	Bowel Prep for MRI	Type of PET/CT	Tracer/ Contrast Agents for PET/CT	Bowel Prep for PET/CT
Kim et al. 2011[88]	None reported	1.5T and 3T magnet, T1 and T2 weighted	None reported	Not reported	FDG	None reported

FDG=[18]F-fluorodeoxyglucose; MRI=magnetic resonance imaging; PET/CT=positron emission tomography/computed tomography.

Table C-24. Reported data: MRI versus PET/CT for rectal staging N

Study, N Patients, Author's Conclusion	Outcomes	MRI Reported N Stage Data	PET/CT Reported N Stage Data	Staging by Pathology	MRI N0	MRI N1+2	PET/CT N0	PET/CT N1+2
Kim et al. 2011[88] 30 patients	Accuracy	83%	70%					
	N0 vs. N1/2 Sensitivity	94%	61%	pN0	8	4	10	2
	Specificity	67%	83%	pN1+2	1	17	7	11
Conclusion: MRI is better								

MRI=magnetic resonance imaging; PET/CT=positron emission tomography/computed tomography.

PET/CT Versus MRI Plus CT

Table C-25. Study design: PET/CT versus MRI+CT

Study	Outcomes Reported	Design	Prospective?	Funded by	Setting	Country	Design
Eglinton et al. 2010[129]	Changes in management–rectal staging	One group (cohort or case series)	Prospective	Not reported	University	Australia	One group (cohort or case series)

Table C-26. Patient details: PET/CT versus MRI+CT

Study	Type of Cancer	Age	% Male
Eglinton et al. 2010[129]	Primary rectal	mean 63, range 45-82	70%

Table C-27. Imaging details: PET/CT versus MRI+CT

Study	MRI+CT Contrast Agents	MRI+CT Type	MRI+CT Bowel Prep	PET/CT Type	PET/CT Tracer/Contrast Agents	PET/CT Bowel Prep
Eglinton et al. 2010[129]	Oral contrast for CT; nothing else reported	Not reported	None reported	Not reported	FDG, oral contrast	None reported

CT=Computed tomography; FDG=^{18}F-fluorodeoxyglucose; MRI=magnetic resonance imaging; PET/CT=positron emission tomography/computed tomography.

Table C-28. Reported data: PET/CT versus MRI+CT for preoperative primary rectal staging changes in management

Study	Type of Cancer, Number of Patients	Design	Results	Conclusions
Eglinton et al. 2009[129]	Primary rectal cancer, 19 patients	Information about the patients (MRI, CT, and clinical information) was sent to another institution where a treatment plan was developed; this was compared with the treatment plan developed in-house using all available information including PET/CT	The addition of PET/CT information led to changes in management in 5 patients; most of these patients were stage 1V. 2 patients would have avoided further investigation of liver lesions, 2 would have undergone further investigation of possible prostate involvement, and neoadjuvant therapy would have been altered in 4 patients. No changes in surgical management would have occurred.	PET/CT provides additional information to conventional staging, but this information only resulted in minor changes in management.

CT=Computed tomography; IV=intravenous; MRI=magnetic resonance imaging; PET/CT=positron emission tomography/computed tomography.

C-36

PET/CT Versus CT

Table C-29. Study design: CT versus PET/CT

Study	Outcomes	Design	Prospective?	Funded by	Setting	Country
Engledow et al. 2012[128]	Changes in management–colorectal staging	One group (cohort or case series)	Prospective	No Surrender Charitable Trust	University	United Kingdom
Uchiyama et al. 2012[89]	Preoperative colorectal T, N and M staging accuracy	One group (cohort or case series)	Prospective	Not reported	University	Japan
Ramos et al. 2011[19]	Preoperative colorectal M staging accuracy, and changes in management	One group (cohort or case series)	Prospective	Instituto de Salud Carlos III	University	Spain
Orlacchio et al. 2009[90]	Preoperative colorectal M staging accuracy	One group (cohort or case series)	Unclear	Not reported	University	Italy
Lubezky et al. 2007[91]	Preoperative and interim colorectal M staging accuracy	One group (cohort or case series)	Unclear	Not reported	University	Israel

Table C-30. Patient details: PET/CT versus CT

Study	Type of Cancer	Age	% Male
Engledow et al. 2012[128]	Colorectal liver metastases	Median: 63 years (Range: 32–79)	63
Uchiyama et al. 2012[89]	Colon and rectal	Mean: 67.7 years (Range: 29–91)	71
Ramos et al. 2011[19]	Colorectal liver metastases	Mean: 63 years (SD: 9.4)	67
Orlacchio et al. 2009[90]	Colorectal liver metastases	Mean: 64.4 years (SD: 10.2)	64.5
Lubezky et al. 2007[91]	Colorectal liver metastases	Mean: 66 years (SD: 9.8)	50%

SD=Standard deviation.

Table C-31. Imaging details: PET/CT versus CT

Study	CT Contrast Agents	CT Type	CT Bowel Prep	PET/CT Type	PET/CT Tracer/Contrast Agents	PET/CT Bowel Prep
Engledow et al. 2012[128]	Not reported	3.75 mm, axial	None	Not reported	FDG, no contrast	None
Uchiyama et al. 2012[89]	Iopamidol 100 ml	2.5mm, helical	None	Not reported	FDG, no contrast	None
Ramos et al. 2011[19]	Nonionic contrast media (2 ml/kg)	1.2 mm, helical	None	Not reported	FDG, no contrast	None
Orlacchio et al. 2009[90]	Nonionic iodinated (Iomeron)	3.75 mm (retrospectively reconstructed to 1.25 mm) slices	None	Not reported	FDG, Gastrografin	None
Lubezky et al. 2007[91]	Iodinated oral contrast	5 mm slices	None	Not reported	FDG, iodinated oral contrast	None

CT=Computed tomography; FDG=^{18}F-fluorodeoxyglucose; kg=kilogram; ml=milliliter; mm=millimeter; PET=positron emission tomography.

Table C-32. Reported data: CT versus PET/CT for colorectal staging T

Study N Patients Author's Conclusions	Outcomes	CT Reported T Stage Data	PET/CT Reported T Stage Data	T Stage by Pathology	CT T1	CT T2	CT T3	CT T4	PET/CT T1	PET/CT T2	PET/CT T3	PET/CT T4
Uchiyama et al. 2012[89] 80 lesions, 77 patients	Accuracy	78.8%	95.0%	pT1	4	NR	NR	NR	11	NR	NR	NR
	T1/T2 vs. T3/T4 Sensitivity	Not reported	Not reported	pT2	NR	8	NR	NR	NR	11	NR	NR
	T1/T2 vs. T3/T4 Specificity	Not reported	Not reported	pT3	NR	NR	44	NR	NR	NR	47	NR
Conclusion: PET/CT is better				pT4	NR	NR	NR	7	NR	NR	NR	7

CT=Computed tomography; NR=not reported; PET=positron emission tomography; PET/CT=positron emission tomography/computed tomography; pT=pathologic tumor stage; T=tumor stage.

Table C-33. Reported data: CT versus PET/CT for colorectal staging N

Study N Patients Author's Conclusion	Outcomes	CT Reported N Stage Data	PET/CT Reported N Stage Data	N Stage by Pathology	CT N0	CT N1+2	PET/CT N0	PET/CT N1+2
Uchiyama et al. 2012[89] 75 patients	Accuracy	70.7%	69.3%					
	Sensitivity N0 vs. N1/2	68.6%	34.3%	pN0	24	11	12	0
	Specificity N0 vs. N1/2	72.5%	100%	pN1+2	11	29	23	40
Conclusion: **CT is better**								

CT=Computed tomography; N=nodal stage; PET=positron emission tomography; pN=pathologic nodal stage.

Table C-34. Reported data: CT versus PET/CT for colorectal staging M

Study N Patients Author's Conclusion	Outcomes	CT Reported M Stage Data	PET/CT Reported M Stage Data
Uchiyama et al. 2012[89] 77 patients (per patient basis)	Accuracy	Not reported	Not reported
	Sensitivity	93.8%	93.8%
	Specificity	Not reported	Not reported
Conclusion: **Equally as good**			
Ramos et al. 2011[19] 70 patients (per lesion basis)	Accuracy	Not reported	Not reported
	Sensitivity	86%[a]	72%[a]
	Specificity	Not reported	Not reported
Conclusion: **CT is better**			
Orlacchio et al. 2009[90] 467 patients (per lesion basis)	Accuracy	92.3%	97.9%
	Sensitivity	91.1%	97.9%
	Specificity	95.4%	97.7%
Conclusion: **PET/CT is better**			
Lubezky et al. 2007[91] 27 patients (per patient basis)	Accuracy	Not reported	Not reported
	Sensitivity	87.5%[a]	93.3%[a]
	Specificity	Not reported	Not reported
Conclusion: **PET/CT is better**			

[a] For the patients who did not have neoadjuvant therapy

CT=Computed tomography; M=metastases stage; PET=positron emission tomography.

Table C-35. Reported data: CT versus PET/CT for interim colorectal restaging M

Study N Patients Author's Conclusion	Outcomes	CT Reported M Stage Data (per Patient Basis)	PET/CT Reported M Stage Data (per Patient Basis)
Lubezky et al. 2007[91]	Accuracy	Not reported	Not reported
48 patients	Sensitivity	65.3%	49%
Conclusion: **CT is better**	Specificity	75%	83.3%

CT=Computed tomography; M=metastases stage; PET=positron emission tomography.

Table C-36. Reported data: CT versus PET/CT for preoperative colorectal staging changes in management

Study	Type of Cancer, Number of Patients	Design	Results	Conclusions
Engledow et al. 2011[128]	Colorectal, 64	Patients referred for evaluation of colorectal metastases were examined by CT and by PET/CT; patient management plans were developed based on CT and clinical factors, and then PET/CT information was revealed and a new plan developed.	Including PET/CT results upstaged disease in 31% and downstaged disease in 3%. Management changed in 34% of patients after adding PET/CT results.	The addition of PET/CT lead to management changes in over a third of patients.
Ramos et al. 2011[19]	Colorectal, 97	Patients referred for evaluation of colorectal metastases were examined by CT and PET/CT; 11 patients also underwent MRI. A treatment plan based on CT and clinical information was developed; then PET/CT information was revealed and a new plan developed. The accuracy of the treatment plans were confirmed by surgical results or 6-month clinical followup.	The addition of PET/CT results changed management in 17.5% of patients, but it turns out the change was the correct choice in only half of these patients- in the other half, the change in management was incorrect and potentially harmful.	PET/CT provided useful information in 8% of cases, and provided incorrect potentially harmful information in 9% of cases.

CT=Computed tomography; MRI=magnetic resonance imaging; PET=positron emission tomography.

MRI Versus CT

Table C-37. Study design: MRI versus CT

Study	Outcomes Reported	Design	Prospective?	Funded by	Setting	Country
Berger-Kulemann et al. 2012[200]	Interim colorectal M restaging accuracy	One group (cohort or case series)	Prospective	Not reported but no COI	University	Austria
Kulemann et al. 2011[201]	Interim colorectal M restaging accuracy	One group (cohort or case series)	Retrospective	Not reported	University	Austria
van Kessel et al. 2011[202]	Interim colorectal M restaging accuracy	One group (cohort or case series)	Prospective	Not reported	University	The Netherlands
Taylor et al. 2007[119]	Preoperative rectal CRM status	One group (cohort or case series)	Retrospective	Not reported	University	United Kingdom
Arii et al. 2006[117]	Preoperative rectal N staging accuracy	One group (cohort or case series)	Prospective	Not reported	University	Japan
Bartolozzi et al. 2004[120]	Preoperative colorectal M staging accuracy	One group (cohort or case series)	Prospective	Not reported	University-based	Italy
Bhattacharjya et al. 2004[121]	Preoperative colorectal M staging accuracy	One group (cohort or case series)	Prospective	Not reported	University-based	United Kingdom
Bohm et al. 2004[122]	Preoperative colorectal M staging accuracy	One group (cohort or case series)	Unclear	Not reported	University-based	Germany
Matsuoka et al. 2003[112]	Preoperative rectal T and N staging accuracy	One group (cohort or case series)	Prospective	Not reported	University-based	Japan
Blomqvist et al. 2002[115]	Pre-radiochemotherapy rectal T staging and interim restaging accuracy	One group (cohort or case series)	Retrospective	Grants from European College of Radiology	University-based	Sweden
Lencioni et al. 1998[123]	Preoperative colorectal M staging accuracy	One group (cohort or case series)	Prospective	Not reported	University-based	Italy

Table C-37. Study design: MRI versus CT (continued)

Study	Outcomes Reported	Design	Prospective?	Funded by	Setting	Country
Strotzer et al. 1997[124]	Preoperative colorectal M staging accuracy	One group (cohort or case series)	Prospective	Not reported	University-based	Germany
Guinet et al. 1990[113]	Preoperative rectal T and N staging accuracy	One group (cohort or case series)	Unclear	Not reported	University-based	France
Hodgman et al. 1986[114]	Preoperative rectal and T and N staging accuracy	One group (cohort or case series)	Unclear	Not reported	Mayo Clinic	U.S.

Table C-38. Patient details: MRI versus CT

Study	Type of Cancer	Age	% Male
Berger-Kulemann et al. 2012[200]	Colorectal liver metastases, with fatty liver	Mean: 62 years (Range: 48–82)	56%
Kulemann et al. 2011[201]	Colorectal liver metastases, with fatty liver	Mean: 64 years (Range: 52–77)	60%
van Kessel et al. 2011[202]	Colorectal liver metastases	Mean: 60.1 (Range: 48–71)	33%
Taylor et al. 2007[119]	Primary rectal	Median: 74 years (Range: 47–93)	Not reported
Arii et al. 2006[117]	Lower rectal	Mean: 62 years (Range: 34–83)	74%
Bartolozzi et al. 2004[120]	Colorectal liver metastases	Not reported	Not reported
Bhattacharjya et al. 2004[121]	Colorectal liver metastases	Median: 62 (Range: 29–74)	53%
Bohm et al. 2004[122]	Colorectal liver metastases	Not reported	Not reported
Matsuoka et al. 2003[112]	Locally advanced rectal	Mean: 64.3 years (Range: 37–83)	66.6%
Blomqvist et al. 2002[115]	Locally advanced rectal	Median: 60 years (Range: 28–76)	62.5%
Lencioni et al. 1998[123]	Colorectal liver metastases	Mean: 58.2 years (Range: 43–76)	61%
Strotzer et al. 1997[124]	Colorectal adenocarcinoma	Mean: 63 years (Range: 32–83)	62.8%
Guinet et al. 1990[113]	Primary rectal (lower and middle)	Mean: 66 years (Range: 49–78)	73.6%
Hodgman et al. 1986[114]	Rectal carcinoma	Range: 35–87 years	58.8%

C-43

Table C-39. Imaging details: MRI versus CT

Study	MRI Contrast Agents	MRI Type	MRI Bowel Prep	CT Type	CT Contrast Agents	CT Bowel Prep
Berger-Kulemann et al. 2012[200]	Gadoxetic acid-enhanced	3.0T magnet, T1 and T2 weighted	No	0.6 mm, axial, reconstructed to 3 mm slices	Nonionic	No
Kulemann et al. 2011[201]	Gd-EOB-GDTP	1.5T 13 patients), 3T (7 patients) magnets, T1 and T2 weighted	No	3 mm slices	Nonionic	No
van Kessel et al. 2011[202]	Gadovist	1.5T magnet, T2 weighted	None reported	5- and 2-mm, helical	Telebrix Gastro (oral), Iopromide (Ultravist) IV	None reported
Taylor et al. 2007[119]	None	1.5T magnet, T1 and T2 weighted, phased-array coil	No	5 mm helical	Intravenous contrast	None reported
Arii et al. 2006[117]	None	1.5T magnet, T1 and T2 weighted, phased-array coil	No	10 mm spiral	Iopromid (300 mg I/ml)	None
Bartolozzi et al. 2004[120]	Not reported	0.5T (n=8), 1.0T (n=6), 1.5T (n=30) magnets, T1 and T2 weighted	None reported	Not reported	Not reported	None reported
Bhattacharjya et al. 2004[121]	Gadolinium, Gadolinium (Dotarem)	1.5T and 1.0T magnets, T1 weighted, body coil	No	7-10 mm, helical	Omnipaque	No
Bohm et al. 2004[122]	Gadolinium chelate (Magnevist)	1.5T magnet, T1 and T2 weighted, body coil	None reported	7.5 mm helical	Oral Peritrast, I.V. Ultravist	None reported
Matsuoka et al. 2003[112]	Air in the rectum, gadolinium (Magnevist)	1.5T magnet, T1 and T2 weighted	Laxative and enema	5 mm slices	Air in the rectum, IV iopamidol (Iopamiron)	Laxative and enema
Blomqvist et al. 2002[115]	IV gadolinium-DTPA-dimeglumine	1.5T magnet, T1 and T2 weighted, phased-array pelvic coil	No	10 mm slices	Oral and IV contrast medium	No

Table C-39. Imaging details: MRI versus CT, (continued)

Study	MRI Contrast Agents	MRI Type	MRI Bowel Prep	CT Type	CT Contrast Agents	CT Bowel Prep
Lencioni et al. 1998[123]	None	1.5T magnet, T1 and T2 weighted, body coil	No	7 mm, helical	Nonionic	None reported
Strotzer et al. 1997[124]	None	1.5T magnet, T1 and T2 weighted, body coil	Not	5 mm, helical	IV iopamideol (Solutrast 300)	No
Guinet et al. 1990[113]	Not reported	0.5T magnet, T1 and T2 weighted	No	Not reported	IV, oral and rectal	No
Hodgman et al. 1986[114]	Air in the rectum	0.15T magnet, weighting not reported, elliptical coil	No	10 mm axial	Oral, IV iodinated contrast medium, and dilute rectal contrast media (Gastrografin)	No

CT=Computed tomography; IV=intravenous; MRI=magnetic resonance imaging.

Table C-40. Reported data: CT versus MRI for preoperative rectal staging T

Study N Patients Author's Conclusion	Outcomes	CT Reported T Stage Data	MRI Reported T Stage Data	T Stage by Pathology	CT T1+T2	CT T3	CT T4	MRI T1+T2	MRI T3	MRI T4
Matsuoka et al. 2003[112] 21 patients	Accuracy	95.2%	100%	pT1+T2	3	1	0	4	0	0
	T1/T2 vs. T3/T4 Sensitivity	100%	100%	pT3	0	15	0	0	15	0
Author's conclusion: **CT was as good as MRI**	T1/T2 vs. T3/T4 Specificity	75%	100%	pT4	0	0	2	0	0	2
Matsuoka et al. 2003[112]	Understaged	0	0							
	Overstaged	1	0							
Guinet et al. 1990[113] 19 patients	Accuracy	94.7%	100%	pT1+pT2	NR	NR	NR	NR	NR	NR
	Understaged	1	0	pT3	NR	NR	NR	NR	NR	NR
Conclusion: **There was no significant difference.**	Overstaged	0	0	pT4	NR	NR	NR	NR	NR	NR
Hodgman et al. 1986[114] 30 had CT of these 27 also had MRI	Accuracy	80%	59%	pT1+pT2	NR	NR	NR	NR	NR	NR
	Understaged	3/30	7/27	pT3	NR	NR	NR	NR	NR	NR
Conclusion: **CT is more accurate**	Overstaged	3/30	4/27	pT4	NR	NR	NR	NR	NR	NR

CT=Computed tomography; MRI=magnetic resonance imaging; NR=not reported; pT=pathologic tumor stage; T=tumor stage.

Table C-41a. Reported data: CT versus MRI for preoperative rectal staging N

Study N Patients Author's Conclusion	Outcomes	CT Reported N Stage Data Regional Lymph Nodes	MRI Reported N Stage Data Regional Lymph Nodes	CT Reported N Stage Data Lateral Pelvic Lymph Nodes	MRI Reported N Stage Data Lateral Pelvic Lymph Nodes
Arii et al. 2006[117] 53 patients Conclusion: **MRI is better**	Accuracy	51%	64%	75%	83%
	N0 vs. N1/2 Sensitivity	50%	71%	33%	56%
	N0 vs. N1/2 Specificity	51%	61%	78%	97%

CT=Computed tomography; MRI=magnetic resonance imaging; N=nodal stage.

Table C-41b. Reported data: CT versus MRI for preoperative rectal staging N

Study N Patients Author's Conclusion	Outcomes	CT Reported N Stage Data	MRI Reported N Stage Data
Matsuoka et al. 2003[112] 21 patients Conclusion: **CT was as good as MRI (data do not support this conclusion)**	Accuracy	62%	71%
	N0 vs. N1/2 Sensitivity	67%	67%
	N0 vs. N1/2 Specificity	58%	75%
Guinet et al. 1990[113] 19 patients Conclusion: **There was no significant difference**	Accuracy	73.7%	73.7%
	Understaged	3/19	4/19
	Overstaged	2/19	1/19
Hodgman et al. 1986[114] 30 patients had CT of these 27 had MRI Conclusion: **CT is better**	Accuracy	65%	39%
	N0 vs. N1/2 Sensitivity	40%	13%
	N0 vs. N1/2 Specificity	90%	88%

CT=Computed tomography; MRI=magnetic resonance imaging; N=nodal stage; pN=pathologic tumor stage.

Table C-42. Reported data: CT versus MRI for preoperative rectal staging CRM status

Study N Patients Author's Conclusion	Outcomes	CT Reported CRM Status Data	MRI Reported CRM Status Data	CRM Status	CT Uni	CT O	MRI Uni	MRI O
Taylor et al. 2007[119]	Accuracy	64.3%	54.8%					
42 patients				pUni	22	11	18	15
	Uni vs. O Sensitivity	55.6%	55.6%	pO	4	5	4	5
	Specificity	66.7%	54.5%					
Conclusion: **Both modalities tended to overstage CRM status; however, they rarely understaged CRM status**								

CRM=Circumferential resection margin; CT=computed tomography; MRI=magnetic resonance imaging; O=CRM is threatened or involved; Uni=Circumferential resection margin is not involved.

Table C-43. Reported data: CT versus MRI for pre-radiochemotherapy rectal staging T

Study N Patients Author's Conclusion	Outcomes	CT Reported T Stage Data	MRI Reported T Stage Data	T Stage Pathology	CT T1	CT T2	CT T3	CT T4	MRI T1	MRI T2	MRI T3	MRI T4
Blomqvist et al. 2002[115]	Accuracy	44.4%	46.2%	pT1	0	0	0	1	0	0	0	1
13 had MRI, and of these, 9 also had CT	T1/T2 vs. T3/T4 Sensitivity	100%	87.5%	pT2	0	0	0	0	0	0	0	0
	T1/T2 vs. T3/T4 Specificity	NR	NR	pT3	0	0	2	0	1	0	0	1
Conclusion: **MRI was not significantly better than CT**				pT4	0	0	4	2	0	0	0	6

CT=Computed tomography; MRI=magnetic resonance imaging; NR=not reported.

Table C-44. Reported data: CT versus MRI for interim rectal restaging T

Study N Patients Author's Conclusion	Outcomes	CT Reported T Stage Data	MRI Reported T Stage Data	T Stage Pathology	CT T1	CT T2	CT T3	CT T4	MRI T1	MRI T2	MRI T3	MRI T4
Blomqvist et al. 2002[115]	Accuracy	41.7%	60.0%	pT1	1	0	1	0	0	0	0	2
15 had MRI, and of these, 12 also had CT	T1/T2 vs. T3/T4 Sensitivity	90.0%	91.7%	pT2	1	0	0	0	1	0	0	0
	T1/T2 vs. T3/T4 Specificity	66.7%	33.3%	pT3	0	0	3	0	1	0	3	1
Conclusion: **MRI was not significantly better than CT**				pT4	1	0	5	1	0	0	1	6

CT=Computed tomography; MRI=magnetic resonance imaging; pT=pathologic tumor stage; T=tumor stage.

Table C-45. Reported data: CT versus MRI for colorectal staging M

Study N Patients Author's Conclusion	Outcomes (per patient basis)	CT Reported M Stage Data (per patient basis)	MRI Reported M Stage Data (per patient basis)	Outcomes (per lesion basis)	CT Reported M Stage Data (per lesion basis)	MRI Reported M Stage Data (per lesion basis)
Bhattacharjya et al. 2004[121]	Accuracy	73%	75.0%	Sensitivity	73.0%	81.9%
100 patients had CT, of these 92 also had MRI	Understaged	15/100	9/92	Specificity	96.5%	93.2%
	Overstaged	12/100	7/92	—	—	—
Conclusion: **The accuracy of both modalities was similar**						
Bohm et al. 2004[122]	—	—	—	Sensitivity	88%	91%
24 patients had CT, of these 23 also had MRI	—	—	—	Specificity	Not calculable	Not calculable
Conclusion: **MRI is better**						
Bartolozzi et al. 2004[120]	Accuracy	50%	50%	Detection rate	71%	72%
44 patients	Understaged	19/44	20/44	—	—	—
	Overstaged	3/44	2/44	—	—	—
Conclusion: **MRI was slightly better**						
Lencioni et al. 1998[123]	—	—	—	Detection rate	21/36 (58%)	19/36 (53%)
14 patients						
Conclusion: **No difference**						
Strotzer et al. 1997[124]	Sensitivity	93%	87%	Detection rate	49%	64%
35 patients	Specificity	95%	95%	False positives	3.9%	3.0%
Conclusion: **CT is better**						

Table C-46. Reported data: CT versus MRI for interim colorectal restaging M

Study		CT Reported M Stage Data (per lesion basis)	MRI Reported M Stage Data (per lesion basis)
Berger-Kulemann et al. 2012[200]	Detection rate	72%	97%
23 patients	False-positives	7 lesions	8 lesions
Conclusion: **MRI is better**			
Kulemann et al. 2011[201]	Detection rate	65%	88%
20 patients	False-positives	1 lesion	0 lesions
Conclusion: **MRI is better**			
Van Kessel et al. 2011[202]	Detection rate	76%	80%
20 patients	False-positives	12 lesions	6 lesions
Conclusion: **MRI is better**			

CT Versus MRI Versus ERUS

Table C-47. Study design: CT versus MRI versus ERUS

Study	Outcomes Reported	Design	Prospective	Funded by	Setting	Country
Martellucci et al. 2012[199]	Interim rectal T and N restaging accuracy	One group (cohort or case series)	Prospective	Not reported	University	Italy
Pomerri et al. 2011[163]	Interim rectal T, N, and CRM status restaging accuracy	One group (cohort or case series)	Prospective	Italian Ministry of Health	University	Italy
Barbaro et al. 1995[92]	Preoperative rectal T staging accuracy	One group (cohort or case series)	Unclear	Not reported	University	Italy

Table C-48. Patient details: CT versus MRI versus ERUS

Study	Type of Cancer	Age	% Male
Martellucci et al. 2012[199]	Locally advanced rectal	Mean: 65.5 years (Range: 45–82)	73%
Pomerri et al. 2011[163]	Primary rectal	Median: 61 years (Range: 20–81)	61%
Barbaro et al. 1995[92]	Primary rectal	Not reported	69%

Table C-49. Imaging details: MRI versus CT versus ERUS

Study	Contrast Agents for MRI	Type of MRI	Bowel Prep for MRI	Type of CT	Contrast Agents for CT	Bowel Prep for CT	Type of ERUS	MHz, ERUS	Bowel Prep for ERUS
Martellucci et al. 2012[199]	Not reported	Not reported	Not reported	Not reported	Not reported	Not reported	Not reported	Not reported	Enema
Pomerri et al. 2011[163]	Gadolinium	1.0T magnet, T1 and T2 weighted, phased-array surface coil	Enema	3 mm helical	IV contrast medium (Ominpaque 350)	Enema	Rotating radial	5–10	Enema
Barbaro et al. 1995[92]	Not reported	Not reported	Not reported	Not reported	Not reported	Not reported	Not reported	Not reported	Not reported

Table C-50. Reported data: CT versus MRI versus ERUS rectal cancer staging T

Study, N Patients, Authors Conclusions		CT Reported T Stage Data	MRI Reported T Stage Data	ERUS Reported T Stage Data
Barbaro et al. 1995[92] 13 patients	Accuracy	61%	66%	90%
Conclusion: **ERUS is better**				

Table C-51. Reported data: CT versus MRI versus ERUS interim rectal restaging T

Study, N Patients, Authors Conclusions		CT Reported T Stage Data	MRI Reported T Stage Data	ERUS Reported T Stage Data
Martellucci et al. 2012[199] 37 patients	Accuracy	59.5%	60.0%	67.5%
	Sensitivity for T2	42.8%	40.0%	28.5%
	Specificity for T2	73.3%	73.3%	93.3%
	Sensitivity for T3	79.1%	83.3%	95.8%
	Specificity for T3	46.1%	46.1%	76.9%
Conclusion: **ERUS is better**				
Pomerri et al. 2011[163] 90 patients	Accuracy	37%	34%	27%
	Understaged	15%	24%	31%
	Overstaged	48%	43%	42%
Conclusion: **All were inaccurate**				

Table C-52. Reported data: CT versus MRI versus ERUS interim rectal restaging N

Study, N patients, Authors Conclusions	Outcomes	CT Reported N Stage Data	MRI Reported N Stage Data	ERUS Reported N Stage Data
Martellucci et al. 2012[199] 37 patients	Accuracy	56.5%	55.0%	75.5%
	Sensitivity	62.5%	50.0%	37.5%
	Specificity	55.1%	55.5%	86.2%
Authors conclusion: **ERUS is better**				
Pomerri et al. 2011[163] 90 patients	Accuracy	62%	68%	65%
	Understaged	6%	15%	18%
	Overstaged	32%	18%	17%
Authors conclusion: **None were accurate**				

Table C-53. Reported data: CT versus MRI versus ERUS interim rectal restaging CRM status

Study, N Patients, Authors Conclusions	Outcome	CT CRM Status	MRI CRM Status	ERUS CRM Status
Pomerri et al. 2011[163] 86 patients	Accuracy	71%	85%	Not applicable
	Specificity	74%	88%	Not applicable
Authors conclusion: **MRI can accurately identify a tumor-free CRM**				

Factors Affecting Individual Modalities

Endorectal Ultrasound

Table C-54. Study design: factors affecting ERUS accuracy

Study	Outcomes Reported	Design	Prospective?	Funded by	Setting	Country
Kim et al. 2004[186]	Impact of water installation on rectal cancer T staging accuracy	One group (cohort or case series)	Prospective	Not reported	University	Korea
Mo et al. 2002[165]	Miniprobe vs. conventional probe for colorectal T and N staging accuracy	Two groups (controlled comparative)	Prospective	Not reported	Community	Taiwan
Hunerbein et al. 2000[187]	3D vs. 2D for rectal cancer T and N staging	One group (cohort or case series)	Unclear	Not reported	University	Germany

Table C-55. Patient details: ERUS factors

Study	Type of Cancer	Age	% Male
Kim et al. 2004[186]	Rectal cancer	Mean 56 (Range: 23 to 91)	49.2%
Mo et al. 2002[165]	A mix of colon and rectal; 57% of the miniprobe group had rectal, 81% of the conventional probe group had rectal	Mean: 63 (Range: 39 to 89)	57% miniprobe group; 48% conventional group
Hunerbein et al. 2000[187]	Rectal adenoma (9 patients), adenocarcinoma (21 patients)	Mean: 65 (Range: 39 to 77)	60%

Table C-56. Imaging details: ERUS factors

Study	Type of ERUS	MHz, ERUS	Bowel Prep, ERUS
Kim et al. 2004[186]	Rigid radial mechanical rotating	7 to 10	Rectal suppository
Mo et al. 2002[165]	Balloon sheath miniprobe, or a lateral viewing conventional probe	12 MHz miniprobe, 7.5 MHz conventional	Rectum filled with water during imaging
Hunerbein et al. 2000[187]	Rigid 3D	10 MHz	None reported

Table C-57. Reported data: factors affecting ERUS for preoperative colorectal staging

Study	Type of Cancer, Number of Patients	Reference Standard	Reported T Stage Data Factors	Reported N Stage Data Factors	Reported M Stage Factors
Kim et al. 2004[186]	Primary rectal, 63	Histopathology	Water instillation during ERUS improves the depiction and local staging of the tumors. Only 67% of the tumors were clearly visible pre-water vs. 100% with water. The accuracy of staging pre-water was 57.1% vs. 85.7% with water.	Not reported	Not reported
Mo et al. 2002[165]	Miniprobe group: 35 rectal, 26 colon; conventional group: 59 rectal, 14 colon	Histopathology	The miniprobe had an overall accuracy of 85%, with an accuracy of 100% for T1, 78% for T2, 90% in T3 and 40% in T4, vs. for conventional probe overall accuracy was 89%, with an accuracy of 83% for T1, 83% for T2, 93% for T3, and 71% for T4.	The miniprobe had a sensitivity of 56% and specificity of 75% for lymph node detection vs. for the conventional probe sensitivity was 77% and specificity was 76%.	Not reported
Hunerbein et al. 2000[187]	Rectal cancer, 30 with conventional ERUS, 25 of these also with 3D ERUS	Histopathology	The accuracy of ERUS for predicting tumor invasion was 84% vs. 88% for 3D ERUS. Both modalities overstaged one patient (the same patient), and ERUS understaged 3 patients vs. 2 patients understaged by 3D ERUS.	This data was discrepant- what was reported in the abstract, what does not match what was reported in the text and the data in the text doesn't have the correct number of patients	Not reported

C-55

Computed Tomography

Table C-58. Study design: factors affecting CT accuracy

Study	Outcomes Reported	Design	Prospective?	Funded by?	Setting	Country
Wicherts et al. 2011[191]	Accuracy of arterial, equilibrium, and venous phase CT for colorectal M staging	One group (cohort or case series)	Unclear	Not reported	University	Netherlands
Lupo et al. 1996[190]	Impact of water enema on CT accuracy for rectal T staging	Two groups (controlled comparative)	Unclear	Not reported	University	Italy
Skriver et al. 1992[189]	Impact of IV contrast on CT accuracy for rectal T and N staging	One group (cohort or case series)	Unclear	Not reported	University	Denmark

Table C-59. Patient details: CT factors

Study	Type of Cancer	Age	% Male
Wicherts et al. 2011[191]	Colorectal cancer liver metastases	Median: 61.9 years (Range: 32.9–83.4)	76%
Lupo et al. 1996[190]	Rectal	Median: 68 years (Range: 30–76)	54.50%
Skriver et al. 1992[189]	Rectal	Median: 65 years (Range: 35–85)	45.40%

Table C-60. Reported data: factors affecting CT for preoperative colorectal staging

Study	Type of Cancer, Number of Patients	Reference Standard	Reported T Stage Data Factors	Reported N Stage Data Factors	Reported M Stage Factors
Wicherts et al. 2011[191]	Colorectal, 53	Intraoperative palpation + ultrasound, and histopathology of resected lesions	Not reported	Not reported	Arterial and equilibrium phase CT have no incremental value compared with hepatic venous phase CT in the detection of liver metastases. Interobserver agreement was 86%.
Lupe et al. 1996[190]	Rectal cancer, 121 total; 37 had water enema, and 64 had standard preparation	Histopathology	Water enema CT was more accurate than standard CT, water enema had an accuracy of 84.2% vs. 62.5% for standard CT	Not reported	Not reported
Skriver et al. 1992[189]	Rectal cancer, 22; all were scanned without IV contrast, immediately after IV contrast, and 10 minutes after IV contrast	Histopathology	There was no difference in accuracy across the 3 different CT procedures; IV contrast media is superfluous for staging rectal cancer	There was no difference in accuracy across the 3 different CT procedures	Not reported

C-57

Magnetic Resonance Imaging

Table C-61. Study design: factors affecting MRI accuracy

Study	Outcomes Reported	Design	Prospective?	Funded by	Setting	Country
Macera et al. 2013[204]	Compared accuracy of T1, T2, contrast-enhanced and diffusion-weighted MRI for interim colorectal M re-staging	One group (cohort or case series)	Retrospective	Not reported	General hospital	Italy
Koh et al. 2012[192]	Compared accuracy of T1, T2, and diffusion-weighted MRI for colorectal M staging	One group (cohort or case series)	Retrospective	Royal Marsden NHS Foundation	University	United Kingdom
Lambregts et al. 2011[203]	Compared accuracy of T2 and diffusion-weighted MRI for rectal N staging	One group (cohort or case series)	Prospective	Not reported	University	The Netherlands
Jao et al. 2010[193]	Compared accuracy of contrast-enhanced and not for rectal T and N staging	One group (cohort or case series)	Retrospective	Not reported	University	Taiwan
Kim et al. 2010[229]	Compared 2D and 3D MRI accuracy for rectal T and N staging	One group (cohort or case series)	Retrospective	Government health ministry	University	South Korea
Futterer et al. 2008[197]	Compared 2D and 3D MRI accuracy for rectal T staging	One group (cohort or case series)	Prospective	Not reported	University	Netherlands
Vliegen et al. 2005[194]	Compared T1 and T2 weighted MRI for rectal T staging	One group (cohort or case series)	Retrospective	Not reported	University	The Netherlands
Kim et al. 2004[196]	Impact of water instillation on rectal T and N staging	One group (cohort or case series)	Unclear	Yonsei University Research Fund	University	South Korea
Okizuka et al. 1996[195]	Compared accuracy of contrast-enhanced and not for rectal T and N staging	One group (cohort or case series)	Prospective	Not reported	University	Japan

Table C-62. Patient details: MRI factors

Study	Type of Cancer	Age	% Male
Macera et al. 2013[204]	Colorectal liver metastases	Median: 65 years (Range: 45–78)	75%
Koh et al. 2012[192]	Colorectal liver metastases	Mean: 64.4 years (Range: 46–78)	61%
Lambregts et al. 2011[203]	Locally advanced rectal	Median: 71 years (Range: 47–90)	83
Jao et al. 2010[193]	Rectal	Mean age: 65 years (Males), Mean age: 64 years (Females)	60%
Kim et al. 2010[229]	Rectal	Mean: 58.4 years (SD: 11.6) (Range: 29–81)	62
Futterer et al. 2008[197]	Rectal	Mean age: 63 years (Range: 33–79)	Not reported
Vliegen et al. 2005[194]	Primary operable rectal	Mean: 64 years (Range: 15–85) Males, Mean: 66 years (Range: 36–86) Females	73
Kim et al. 2004[196]	Rectal	Mean: 56 years (Range: 2–80)	67.7
Okizuka et al. 1996[195]	Rectal	Mean: 65 years (Range: 45–85)	78

Table C-63. Imaging details: MRI factors

Study	Type	Contrast Agents	Bowel Prep
Macera et al. 2013[204]	1.5T magnet, T1, T2, and diffusion-weighting	Intravenous Gd-EOB-DTPA	No
Koh et al. 2012[192]	1.5T magnet, T1, T2, and diffusion-weighting	Intravenous Gd-EOB-DTPA	Not reported
Lambregts et al. 2011[203]	1.5T, T2 and diffusion-weighting, phased-array body coil	None	Not reported
Jao et al. 2010[193]	1.5T, T1 and T2 weighting, phased-array cardiac coil	Gadolinium	No
Kim et al. 2010[229]	3T, T2 weighting, phased-array surface coil	No	No
Futterer et al. 2008[197]	3T, T2 weighting, 3D and 2D, phased-array surface coil	Warm ultrasound gel in rectum	No
Vliegen et al. 2005[194]	1.5T, T1 and T2 weighting, phased-array spine coil	Gadolinium	No
Kim et al. 2004[196]	1.5T, T1 and T2 weighting, phased-array body coil	Warm water in rectum	No
Okizuka et al. 1996[195]	1.5T, T1 and T2 weighting, body coil (17 patients), phased-array coil (15 patients)	Double-contrast barium enema, air in rectum, IV gadopentetate	Glycerin enema

Table C-64. Reported data: factors affecting MRI for colorectal staging

Study	Type of Cancer, Number of Patients	Reference Standard	Reported T Stage Data Factors	Reported N Stage Data Factors	Reported M Stage Factors
Macera et al. 2013[204]	Colorectal, interim re-staging, 32 patients	Intraoperative ultrasound, and histopathology	Not reported	Not reported	Contrast-enhanced MRI, with or without the addition of diffusion-weighted MRI were performed to detect liver metastases. Combining all of the modalities had the highest accuracy (148 of 166 lesions) with a sensitivity for malignancy of 91%.
Koh et al. 2012[192]	Colorectal, 72	Surgical findings and patient followup	Not reported	Not reported	Diffusion-weighted MRI and contrast-enhanced gadolinium-ethoxybenzyl-diethylenetriaminepentaacetic acid (Gd-EOB-DTPA) T1 and T2 weighted MRI were performed to detect liver metastases. 417 lesions were identified. Combing all of the images yielded the highest accuracy, diffusion-weighted MRI was slightly more accurate than contrast-enhanced T1/T2 weighted MRI.

C-61

Table C-64. Reported data: factors affecting MRI for colorectal staging (continued)

Study	Type of Cancer, Number of Patients	Reference Standard	Reported T Stage Data Factors	Reported N Stage Data Factors	Reported M Stage Factors
Lambregts et al. 2011[203]	Rectal cancer, interim restaging, 30 patients	Histopathology	Not reported	T2 and diffusion-weighted MRI were performed on all patients after neoadjuvant chemoradiation and before surgery. T2 had a sensitivity of 65%, specificity of 93%; diffusion-weighted MRI could not distinguish between malignant and benign nodes.	Not reported
Jao et al. 2010[193]	Rectal cancer, 37 patients	Histopathology	All patients underwent T2-weighted and gadolinium-enhanced T1 weighted MRI. Adding contrast-enhanced MRI to the T2 imaging protocol did not improve staging accuracy.	All patients underwent T2-weighted and gadolinium-enhanced T1 weighted MRI. Adding contrast-enhanced MRI to the T2 staging protocol did not improve nodal staging accuracy.	Not reported
Kim et al. 2010[197]	Rectal cancer, 109 patients	Histopathology	All patients underwent T2-weighted 2D and 3D MRI. Accuracy of T stage did not differ between the two modalities, but tumor conspicuity was better on 2D.	All patients underwent T2-weighted 2D and 3D MRI. Accuracy of N stage did not differ between the two modalities.	Not reported
Futterer et al. 2008[197]	Rectal cancer, 22 patients	Histopathology	All patients underwent T2-weighted 2D and 3D MRI. There were significantly more motion artifacts on 3D. Accuracy for T2 was 95% for 2D and 89% for 3D; accuracy for T3 was 86% for 2D and 77% for 3D.	Not reported	Not reported
Vliegen et al. 2004[194]	Rectal cancer, 83 patients	Histopathology	All patients underwent T2 weighted MRI and gadolinium-enhanced T1 weighted MRI. Adding the contrast-enhanced T1 MRI to the T2 MRI did not improve the accuracy of assessing T stage over T2 alone.	Not reported	Not reported

C-62

Table C-64. Reported data: factors affecting MRI for colorectal staging (continued)

Study	Type of Cancer, Number of Patients	Reference Standard	Reported T Stage Data Factors	Reported N Stage Data Factors	Reported M Stage Factors
Kim et al. 2004[196]	Rectal cancer, 62 patients	Histopathology	All patients underwent T1 and T2 weighted imaging before and after filling the rectum with warm water. The water-filled images were more accurate in T staging.	All patients underwent T1 and T2 weighted imaging before and after filling the rectum with warm water. The water did not affect N stage accuracy.	Not reported
Okizuka et al. 1996[195]	Rectal cancer, 32 patients	Histopathology	All patients underwent conventional T1 and T2 weighted MRI, and also gadopentetate dimeglumine enhanced fat-suppressed MRI imaging. Conventional imaging had an accuracy of T staging of 72%, and contrast-enhanced the accuracy was 68%. Contrast-enhanced imaging overstaged 12 patients, while conventional imaging overstaged 9 patients. The accuracy of staging was not improved by using contrast-enhanced imaging.	All patients underwent conventional T1 and T2 weighted MRI, and also gadopentetate dimeglumine enhanced fat-suppressed MRI imaging. Contrast-enhanced imaging was not useful for N staging.	Not reported

C-63

Harms, Device Failure, and Adverse Events

Table C-65. Adverse events reported by included studies from CT, ERUS, and MRI staging

Study	Number of Patients	Cancer Type	Modality	CT Harms	ERUS Harms	ERUS Probe Specifics	MRI Harms
Pomerri et al. 2011[163]	53	Locally advanced rectal	CT ERUS MRI	None reported	Transducer not tolerated in 5 patients, refused by 2 patients	Rotating	7 patients declined MRI due to claustrophobia
Huh et al. 2008[164]	60 had ERUS, and 80 had CT	Locally advanced rectal, within 7 cm from the anal verge	CT ERUS	23 patients refused or experienced pain during CT or ERUS exam	23 patients refused or experienced pain during CT or ERUS exam	Rubber sheath, 360 rotating	Not applicable
Bhattacharjya et al. 2004[121]	85	Colorectal with liver metastases (some suspected)	CT MRI	None reported	Not applicable	Not applicable	13 patients declined MRI due to claustrophobia
Brown et al. 2004[125]	54	Primary rectal	ERUS MRI	Not applicable	11 patients experienced severe pain or declined the procedure	Radial scanning	Not reported
Milsom et al. 1992[118]	14	Recurrent rectal	CT ERUS	None reported	Median VAS for degree of discomfort: 3 (10 representing maximal pain)	Not reported	Not applicable
Rifkin et al. 1986[109]	71	Primary rectal	CT ERUS	None reported	7 patients had minor bleeding	Radial and linear, at least 25 cm long	Not applicable
Rifkin et al. 1986[110]	51	Primary rectal	CT ERUS	None reported	2 patients had minor bleeding, mild discomfort was experienced by all	Not reported	Not applicable

CM=Centimeters; CT=computed tomography; ERUS=endorectal ultrasonography.

Table C-66. Device failures

Study	Number of Patients	Cancer Type	Imaging Modalities	CT Failures	ERUS Failures	MRI Failures
Starck et al. 1995[96]	34	Rectal	MRI ERUS	Not applicable	A malignant stricture prevented passage of the ERUS in 1 (2.9%) patient	No
Mo et al. 2002[165]	134 73 had conventional ERUS, 61 had miniprobe ERUS	A mix of colon and rectal; 81% of the conventional had rectal, 57% of the miniprobe had rectal	ERUS	Not applicable	Failure in 8 (11%) of the conventional group and 2 (3.3%) of the miniprobe group due to stenosis or sharp angulations making visibility difficult	Not applicable
Thaler et al. 1994[97]	37	Primary rectal	MRI ERUS	Not applicable	2 (5.4%) failures due to stenosis	No tumor could be visualized in 1 (2.7%) patient.
Fleshman et al. 1992[116]	19	Advanced rectal	CT ERUS	No tumor could be visualized in 1 (5.2%) patient.	None reported	Not applicable
Goldman et al. 1991[103]	30	Rectal cancer within 10 cm of the anal verge	CT ERUS	No tumor could be visualized in 1 (3.3%) patient.	None reported	Not applicable
Rotte et al. 1989[105]	30	Primary rectal	CT ERUS	None reported	5 (17%) failures. The transducer could not pass due to a tight stenosis in 3 patients, lesions were unreachable due to the short range of the transducer in 2 patients.	Not applicable
Kramann et al. 1986[108]	30	Primary rectal	CT ERUS	Technical failure of the scanner in one exam.	None reported	Not applicable

CT=Computed tomography; ERUS=endorectal ultrasonography; MRI=magnetic resonance imaging

Table C-67. MRI-related adverse events

Study	Study Design	Number of Patients	Diagnosis	Age, Years (Mean±SD)	% Male	N Harmed (%)	Adverse Events	Notes
Semelka et al. 2013[150]	Proof-of-concept	59	Patients with orders for brain or abdominal MRI scans	52 (Range: 5–85)	52.5	0	Not applicable	Setting: Department of Radiology at a U.S. university hospital Timing: NR CA: gadobutrol (Gadavist; Bayer) vs. gadobenate dimeglumine (MultiHance; Bracco)
Albiin et al. 2012[151]	Efficacy	31 31 patients received 0.8 g and 0.4 g, 30 patients received 0.2 g	Healthy	24.3 (Range: 18–48)	56.2%	≥1 AE: 25 (80.6%) at 0.8 g, 18 (58.1%) at 0.4 g, and 10 (33.3%) at 0.2 g ≥1 ADR: 22 (71.0%) at 0.8 g, 13 (41.9%) at 0.4 g, and 7 (23.3%) at 0.2 g	Mild ADRs/AEs: 32 at 0.8 g, 14 at 0.4 g, 6 at 0.2g Moderate ADRs/AEs: 6 at 0.8 g, 1 at 0.4 g, 1 at 0.2 g Severe ADRs/AEs: 1 at 0.8 g, 1 at 0.2 g Most common ADRs were diarrhea, nausea, headache and fatigue.	Setting: University hospital, Sweden Timing: Feb. to May 2010 CA: manganese chloride tetrahydrate (CMC-001) "Liver MRI using 0.8 g CMC-001 has the highest efficacy and still acceptable ADRs and should therefore be preferred."

Table C-67. MRI-related adverse events

Study	Study Design	Number of Patients	Diagnosis	Age, Years (Mean±SD)	% Male	N Harmed (%)	Adverse Events	Notes
Bredart et al. 2012[152]	Prospective, non-randomized, multicenter	365	At risk for breast cancer	59.1% <50 years, 26.9% 50–59 years, 14% ≥60	0	NR	Significant MRI discomfort was due to immobility (37.5%), lying in the tunnel (20.6%), noise of the machine (64.6%), or panic feelings during MRI (6.1%).	Setting: 21 cancer centers, teaching hospitals, or private clinics in France Timing: Nov. 2006 to June 2008

C-67

Table C-67. MRI-related adverse events, (continued)

Study	Study Design	Number of Patients	Diagnosis	Age, Years (Mean±SD)	% Male	N Harmed (%)	Adverse Events	Notes
Maurer et al. 2012[153]	Post-marketing surveillance	84,621 50% neurological exams, 12.2% internal organs, 32.1% musculoskeletal system, 2.3% MR angiographies, 4.9% not specified	19,354 (22.9%) were considered at risk 11.4% history of allergies, 6.6% hypertension, 2.3% CHD, 1.9% CNS disorders, 1.3% bronchial asthma, 1.3% beta blocker treatment, 1.2% cardiac insufficiency, 0.9% renal failure, 0.8% history of allergic reaction to contrast medium, 1.3% liver dysfunction, 1.3% other	52.0±16.9	45.4	285 (0.34%) 421 AEs	65 different AEs were reported. 10 most common included nausea (0.2%), vomiting (0.1%) and less than 1% of patients had the following symptoms: pruritus, urticaria, dizziness, feeling of warmth, retching, sweating increased, paresthesia, and taste alteration. Serious AEs: 8 (<0.01%) 3 of these patients had life-threatening AEs, 1 of the 3 had inpatient treatment. "A causal relationship with GD-DOTA was considered probable in 1 patient, possible in 4 patients, and doubtful in 3 patients."	Setting: 129 German radiology centers Timing: Jan. 2004 to Jan. 2010 CA: gadoteric acid (Gd-DOTA, Dotarem®), manually injected in 74.5%, automated injection in 25.5% Classification: WHO Adverse Reaction Terminology (1998) Allergies and history of allergic reaction to contrast medium were significantly associated (at 0.001 level) with increased risk of adverse events. Renal failure, liver dysfunction or beta blocker intake were not associated with increased risk of adverse events.

Table C-67. MRI-related adverse events, (continued)

Study	Study Design	Number of Patients	Diagnosis	Age, Years (Mean±SD)	% Male	N Harmed (%)	Adverse Events	Notes
Voth et al. 2011[154]	Integrated retrospective analysis (34 clinical studies)	4,549 received gadobutrol (Gadovist/ Gadavist) 1,844 received comparator contrast agents	Severe renal impairment: 38 gadobutrol, 5 comparator Moderate renal impairment: 328 gadobutrol, 132 comparator Mild renal impairment: 846 gadobutrol, 416 comparator Impaired liver function: 214 gadobutrol, 82 comparator Cardiovascular disease: 1506 gadobutrol, 435 comparator History of allergies: 462 gadobutrol History of allergies to contrast agents: 33 gadobutrol	54.2±16.6 gadobutrol 54.7±14.5 comparator	58.5% gado-butrol 52.7% com-parator	182 (4.0%) gadobutrol-related 74 of 1,844 (4.0%) related to comparators	Serious AEs: 21 17 (0.4%) gadobutrol, 4 (0.2%) comparator Drug-related serious AEs: 1 (<0.1%) gadobutrol	Setting: 55.3% Europe, 7.2% U.S./Canada, 7.7% South/Central America, 29.6% Asia, 0.3% Australia Timing: Trials conducted between 1993 and 2009 CA: gadobutrol (Gadovist/Gadavist); Comparator contrast agents included: gadopentetate dimeglumine (Magnevist, N=912), gadoteridol (ProHance, N=555), gadoversetamide (OptiMark, N=227), or gadodiamide (Omniscan, N=150). Classification: MedDRA v. 12.1 "Gadobutrol was well tolerated by patients with impaired liver or kidney function, and by patients with cardiovascular disease."

Table C-67. MRI-related adverse events, (continued)

Study	Study Design	Number of Patients	Diagnosis	Age, Years (Mean±SD)	% Male	N Harmed (%)	Adverse Events	Notes
Forsting and Palkowitsch 2010[155]	Integrated retrospective analysis (6 clinical studies)	14,299 14.7% MRA	NR	53.7	46.6	78 (0.55%) 82.4% occurred within 5 minutes of administration, 1 patient had an ADR 9 hours post-injection	Serious: 2 (0.01%) gadobutrol-related; 1 severe anaphylactoid reaction, 1 itching/swelling of throat Most frequently reported: nausea (0.25%)	Setting: 300 radiology centers in Europe and Canada Timing: 2000 to 2007 CA: gadobutrol "Gadobutrol 1.0M is well tolerated and has a good safety profile. The occurrence of ADRs observed following the intravenous injection of gadobutrol is comparable with the published data of other Gd-based contrast agents."
Ichikawa et al. 2010[156]	Multicenter, open-label, prospective Phase III	178	Suspected focal hepatic lesions	66 (Range: 31–82)	72.4	44 (24.7%)	Mild: 56 Moderate: 6	Setting: 15 radiology departments in Japan Timing: Aug. 2001 to July 2003 CA: Combined unenhanced and gadoxetic acid disodium (Gd-EOB-DTPA)

Table C-67. MRI-related adverse events, (continued)

Study	Study Design	Number of Patients	Diagnosis	Age, Years (Mean±SD)	% Male	N Harmed (%)	Adverse Events	Notes
Ishiguchi and Takahashi 2010[157]	Post-marketing surveillance	3,444	Liver disorder: 9.52% Kidney disorder: 2.85%	1% <15 years, 58.51% 15 to <65 years, 40.30% ≥65	49.45	32 (0.93%)	Mild: 36 (0.49% gastrointestinal-related disorders most commonly reported) Moderate: 4 2 patients with nausea, 2 with abnormal liver function	Setting: Department of Radiology at a medical university in Japan Timing: March 2001 to March 2005 CA: Gadoterate Meglumine (Gd-DOTA) "Statistically significant risk factors for experiencing adverse reactions were general condition, liver disorder, kidney disorder, complication, concomitant treatments, and Gd-DOTA dose."
Leander et al. 2010[158]	Crossover randomized	18	Healthy	25.0	100	19 AEs	19 mild gastrointestinal	Setting: Swedish university hospital Timing: NR CA: oral Manganese (McCl$_2$)
Hammersting et al. 2009[159]	Multicenter, Phase III, randomized, interindividually controlled comparison	572 292 gado-butrol, 280 gado-pentetate	Patients with known focal lesions of the liver or suspected liver lesions			24 (4.2%) 10 (3.4%) gadobutrol, 21 (5.0%) gadopentetate	4 AEs definitely related to agents, 14 AEs possibly/probably related to agents No serious or severe AEs were reported.	Setting: 25 centers in 8 European countries Timing: NR CA: gadobutrol (Gadovist), gadopentetate (Magnevist)

Table C-67. MRI-related adverse events, (continued)

Study	Study Design	Number of Patients	Diagnosis	Age, Years (Mean±SD)	% Male	N Harmed (%)	Adverse Events	Notes
Shah-Patel et al. 2009[140]	Retrospective chart review	106,800 total 49,731 MRI	NR	Range: 18–86	NR	15 (0.03%)	Mild: 4 Itching or hives Moderate: 6 Vomiting: 3, Lightheaded sensation: 1 Fall: 1, Headache: 1 Severe: 1 Shortness of breath (before examination) Others: 4 Infiltrations at IV site: 2 Mild burns due to contact with magnetic resonance coil during the examination	Setting: Outpatient radiology in New York, NY Timing: over 4 years Total harms: 59 (0.06%) CA: gadopentetate dimeglumine (Magnevist; Berlex) Patients requiring assistance from emergency medical services: 18 (31%)
Schieren et al. 2008[160]	Prospective observational	38	Hemodialysis patients	54.4	63.1	24 (63.1%)	Mild to Moderate: 77 (after 64 MRIs) Severe: 3 One patient developed NSF after undergoing 6 Gd-enhanced MRI studies (5 with Gd-DTPA from August 2004 to January 2005. The patient died of septic complications in March 2006.	Setting: university hospital, Germany Timing: 2003 to 2005 CA: Gd-DTPA, 25 patients also underwent 20 gadobutrol-enhanced MRI and 16 MRIs with 0.9% saline. No AEs were reported.

ADR=Adverse drug event; AE=adverse event; CA=contrast agent; CHD=coronary heart disease; CNS=central nervous system; Gd=Gadolinium; Gd-DTPA=Gd-diethylenetriamine penta-acetic acid; MRA=magnetic resonance angiography; NR=not reported; NSF=nephrogenic systemic fibrosis.

Table C-68. CT-related adverse events

Study	Study Design	Number of Patients	Diagnosis	Age, Years (Mean±SD)	% Male	N Harmed (%)	Adverse Events	Notes
Kim et al. 2013[130]	Prospective cohort	1,048	Renal disease: 20 Cardiovascular disease: 38 Other allergic disease: 91	55.1±14.5	47.8	61 (5.8%)	Immediate reactions: Mild: 51 Moderate: 1 Nonimmediate reaction: Mild: 8 Moderate: 1	Setting: Seoul National University Bundang Hospital, Korea Timing: July to November 2010 Contrast medium (CM): 721 (68.8%) Iopromide, 323 (0.8%) Iomeprol, 3 (0.3%) Iohexol, and 1 (0.1%) Iodixanol "RCM skin testing for screening is of no clinical utility in predicting hypersensitivity reactions."

Table C-68. CT-related adverse events, (continued)

Study	Study Design	Number of Patients	Diagnosis	Age, Years (Mean±SD)	% Male	N Harmed (%)	Adverse Events	Notes
Kobayashi et al. 2013[131]	Retrospective cohort	36,472	Diabetes: 7,138 (19.5%) Hypertension: 10,461 (28.6%) Dyslipidemia: 5,972 (16.4%)	58.3	52	779 (2.1%)	Acute adverse reactions (mild): 756 Nausea/vomiting, rash, coughing/sneezing Severe reactions: 23 Shock, hypotension, desaturation, and airway obstruction	Setting: A community hospital in Tokyo, Japan Timing: April 2004 to March 2011 CM: non-ionic low-osmolar contrast agents such as iopamidol, iohexol, ioversol or iomeprol In multivariate logistic regression analysis, an adverse reaction history to contrast agents, urticaria, allergic history to drugs other than contrast agents, contrast agent concentration >70%, age <50 years, and total contrast agent dose >65 grams were significant predictors of an acute adverse reaction.

C-74

Table C-68. CT-related adverse events, (continued)

Study	Study Design	Number of Patients	Diagnosis	Age, Years (Mean±SD)	% Male	N Harmed (%)	Adverse Events	Notes
Davenport et al. 2012[132]	Retrospective database review	24,826 injections of IV Iopamidol 12,684 injections during warming period, 12,142 injections during no warming		51 (Range: 1–79 years) period 1 52 (Range: 4–90 years), period 2	42% period 1, 28% period 2	177 (0.7%) Warming: 82 No warming: 95	Iopamidol 300 (no warming): 69 Extravasations: 23 Allergic-like reactions: 46 (41 mild, 5 moderate) Iopamidol 300 (warming): 74 Extravasations: 32 Allergic-like reactions: 42 (33 mild, 8 moderate, 1 severe [patient developed pulseless electric activity after injection and although use of CPR returned the patient to normal sinus rhythm, an infected sternotomy wound reopened, and became infected. The patient died 2 months later of complications related to the infected site.]) Iopamidol 370 (no warming): 26 Extravasations: 18 Allergic-like reactions: 8 (6 mild, 2 moderate) Iopamidol 370 (warming): 8 Extravasations: 5 Allergic-like reactions: 3 (all mild)	Setting: Duke University Medical Center, Durham, NC Timing: March 14, 2010 to April 19, 2011 (period 1), October 1, 2010 to April 19, 2011 (period 2) CM: Iopamidol 300 for CT exams, Iopamidol 370 for CT angiographic exams "Extrinsic warming (to 37°C) does not appear to affect adverse event rates for intravenous injections of iopamidol 300 of less than 6 m./sec but is associated with a significant reduction in extravasation and overall adverse event rates for the more viscous iopamidol 370."

Table C-68. CT-related adverse events, (continued)

Study	Study Design	Number of Patients	Diagnosis	Age, Years (Mean±SD)	% Male	N Harmed (%)	Adverse Events	Notes
Jung et al. 2012[144]	Retrospective chart review	47,338	Medical history of 50 patients with cutaneous adverse reactions (CARs): 17 malignant neoplasm, 13 hypertension, 6 diabetes mellitus, 5 allergic history, 5 renal disease, 3 past adverse reactions to contrast medium, 2 tuberculosis, 2 hepatitis	0 to >80 years; focus on CARs occurring in 50 patients (age range: 18 to 81)	58	62 (.13%) 50 (80.7% of overall AEs) CARs	Severe reactions: 16 (25.8% of overall AEs) Dizziness, severe generalized urticaria, hypotension, and facial edema Immediate CARs (46 [92% of CARs]) Urticaria: 39 (78%) Angioedema: 5 (10%) Erythema: 1 (2%) Pruritus without rash: 1 (2%) Delayed CARS (4 [8% of CARs]) Maculopapular rash: 4 (8%)	Setting: Seoul, Korea Timing: Aug. 2005 to Nov. 2009 CM: nonionic monomers including iomeprol, iopamidol, iopromide, and ioversol
Kingston et al. 2012[133]	Prospective cohort	26,854 CT and CTA (50)	Multiple clinical factors and comorbidities	NR	NR	119 (.44%)	Extravasations: 119 (0.44%) 39 (.34%) cannulations performed in the hospital, 80 performed prior Extravasation occurred at the elbow (71.4%), forearm (10.9%), wrist (6.7%) and hand (7.6%).	Setting: a hospital in Australia Timing: Sept. 2004 to April 2008 CM: nonionic IV (Ultravist 300) "Presence of cancer, hypertension, smoking and recent surgery was associated with higher extravasation rates."

C-76

Table C-68. CT-related adverse events, (continued)

Study	Study Design	Number of Patients	Diagnosis	Age, Years (Mean±SD)	% Male	N Harmed (%)	Adverse Events	Notes
Mitchell et al. 2012[134]	Prospective consecutive cohort	633 174 CTPA for PE 459 non-CTPA	**CTPA:** Anemia: 11% DM: 19% History of hypertension: 54% Vascular disease: 15% Congestive heart failure: 12% Baseline renal insufficiency: 10% **Non-CTPA:** Anemia: 13% DM: 17% History of hypertension: 39% Vascular disease: 8% Congestive heart failure: 5% Baseline renal insufficiency: 10%	CTPA: 50±16 Non-CTPA: 46±15	CTPA: 34 Non-CTPA: 46		**CIN:** CTPA: 25 (14%, 95% Confidence Interval: 10% to 20%) Non-CTPA: 45 (9.8%) Severe renal failure: 3 CTPA Death from renal failure: 2 CTPA **All-cause 45-day mortality rate:** 15 CTPA: 6 (3%), death due to renal failure (6), patients with CIN (4) Non-CTPA: 9 (2%)	Setting: a large U.S. academic tertiary care center Timing: June 2007 to January 2009 CM: NR "Development of CIN was associated with an increased risk of death from any cause (relative risk=12, 95% Confidence Interval: 3 to 53)."

Table C-68. CT-related adverse events, (continued)

Study	Study Design	Number of Patients	Diagnosis	Age, Years (Mean±SD)	% Male	N Harmed (%)	Adverse Events	Notes
Vogl et al. 2012[135]	Observational, non-interventional, prospective, multicenter	10,836	5,033 (46.4%) had 1 to 7 concomitant diseases (including DM (6.9%) and renal insufficiency (0.9%) that could potentially influence tolerability of ioversol	60.9	48.1	30 (0.28%)	Mild: 26 Urticaria: 13 Nausea: 11 Erythema: 6 Serious: 4 Anaphylactoid adverse reactions requiring hospitalization: 3 Patients with ≥1 AE: 30	Setting: 72 centers in Germany Timing: August 2006 to April 2007 CM: ioversol
Cadwallader et al. 2011[136]	Prospective audit	198 scans	Pancreatitis: 5.2% Biliary pathology: 11.2% Appendicitis: 12.6% Bowel obstruction: 9% Peptic ulcer disease: 3.2% Diverticular disease: 6.6% Postoperative complications: 3.6% No diagnosis: 13.2% Transferred specialty: 4.6% Other 30.8%	50.4 (Range: 16–94)	44.4	41 (20.7%) scans didn't alter management and were deemed as unnecessarily exposing patients to CT radiation	Risk of fatal cancer induction female aged: 20: 1 in 1,675 30-50: 1 in 2,452 60: 1 in 3,070 70: 1 in 4,113 80: 1 in 7,130 Risk of fatal cancer induction male aged: 30-50: 1 in 2,523 60: 1 in 3,897 80: 1 in 4,289	Setting: Tertiary referral surgical unit Timing: March–May 2008 "The potential diagnostic benefits must outweigh the risks. Figures from the U.S. from 2007 suggest 19,500 CT scans were undertaken each day – the equivalent radiation dose of up to 5,850,000 chest radiographs."

Table C-68. CT-related adverse events, (continued)

Study	Study Design	Number of Patients	Diagnosis	Age, Years (Mean±SD)	% Male	N Harmed (%)	Adverse Events	Notes
Hatakeyama et al. 2011[137]	Retrospective chart review	50 (64 CTAs)	Peritoneal Dialysis	55.0±13.1	68	2 (0.04%)	Mild: 1 Skin disorder Serious: 1 Atrial fibrillation	Setting: A hospital and research institute in Japan Timing: 2002 to 2009 CM: Iopamidol, a low osmolar nonionic
Loh et al. 2010[138]	Prospective surveillance	539 258 iohexol (51 CTA, 209 CT) 281 control (un-enhanced CT)	NR	53.05±14.9	57.7% iohexol 46.9% control	87 (16.1%) 76 (29.4%) iohexol 11 (3.9%) Control	Delayed adverse reactions (DAR): 37 (14.3%) iohexol, 7 (2.5%) control; p<0.0001 Skin rashes or itching: Iohexol: 13 (5.0%), Control: 2 (0.71%); P=0.00273 Patients with cutaneous DARs: Iohexol: 26 (10.1%), Control: 2 (0.71%); P<0.0001 Skin redness (p=0.0055), skin swelling (p=0.0117) and headache (p=0.0246) also occurred statistically more frequently in the iohexol group.	Setting: Tertiary academic medical center Timing: 2006 to 2008 CM: iohexol "This study substantiates a frequent occurrence of DARs at contrast-enhanced CT compared with that in control subjects."

Table C-68. CT-related adverse events, (continued)

Study	Study Design	Number of Patients	Diagnosis	Age, Years (Mean±SD)	% Male	N Harmed (%)	Adverse Events	Notes
Ozbulbul et al. 2010[139]	Prospective	52 MDCT coronary angiography	Suspected coronary artery disease	56.4±13.6 iodixanol (N=28) 54.1±17.1 iopamidol (N=24)	38	32 (61.5%)	Moderate: 32 (61.5%) Intense injection-related heat: Iodixanol: 11 (39.3%) Iopamidol: 20 (83.3%) Nausea: Iodixanol: 1 (3.5%), Iopamidol: 6 (25%) Dizziness: Iodixanol: 0, Iopamidol: 3 (12.5%)	Setting: radiology department, Turkey Timing: Jan. 2008 to June 2008 CM: iopamidol 370 (a low-osmolar) vs. iodixanol 320 (an iso-osmolar) "Iodixanol 320 causes less frequent sensation of heat on intravenous injection. This means more comfort and success in following the breath-hold commands of patients during scanning."
Shah-Patel et al. 2009[140]	Retrospective chart review	106,800 total 33,321 CT	NR	Range: 18–86	NR	35 (0.10%)	Mild: 17 Itching or hives, most often related to iodine-based intravenous contrast injections Moderate: 7 Falls: 3, Nasal congestion: 1, Nausea: 2 Dizziness: 1 Severe: 5 Shortness of breath after IV injection: 5 Others: 6 Infiltrations at IV site: 5, Hematoma at IV site: 1	Setting: Outpatient radiology center in New York, NY Timing: over 4 years CM: iopromide (Ultravist 300)

Table C-68. CT-related adverse events, (continued)

Study	Study Design	Number of Patients	Diagnosis	Age, Years (Mean±SD)	% Male	N Harmed (%)	Adverse Events	Notes
Shie et al. 2008[141]	Prospective	8,776 2,766 Iothala-mate 6,010 Iopromide	Hypertension, diabetes mellitus, asthma, renal disease, heart disease, liver disease, autoimmune disease, and history of allergy	57.0±14.9 Iothalamate 58.2±16.0 Iopromide	NR	127 (1.45%) immediate ADRs 51 (1.84%) Iothalamate 76 (1.26%) Iopromide	Grade I (mild): 21 Iothalamate, 27 Iopromide; p=0.09 Grade II (moderate): 30 Iothalamate, 48 Iopromide; p=0.22 Grade III (severe): 0 Iothalamate, 1 case of Cyanosis, severe laryngeal edema occurred in Iopromide group; p=1.00	Setting: hospital in Taiwan, Republic of China Timing: May 2004 to Dec. 2004 CM: iothalamate meglumine vs iopromide
Weisbord et al. 2008[142]	Prospective cohort of patients scheduled for CT with IV radiocontrast, coronary angiography, or noncoronary angiography	660 total 421 CT	At increased risk for contrast-induced acute kidney injury (CIAKI) Comorbidities: 41 diabetes mellitus, 14 liver disease, 16 congestive heart failure, 13 peripheral vascular disease, and 11 cerebrovascular disease	69±10	96	See incidence	CIAKI: Incidence of CIAKI based on relative increases in SCr levels: ≥25: 6.5 ≥50: 0.5 ≥100: 0.0 Incidence based on absolute changes in SCr levels: ≥0.25 mg/dL: 10.9 ≥0.5 mg/dL: 3.5 ≥1.0 mg/dL: 0.3 Serious: 10 Death 30 days post-CT: 10	Setting: Veterans Affairs Pittsburgh Health System; 25 inpatient, 70 ambulatory, 5 long-term care CT procedures Timing: Feb. 2005 to July 31, 2006 CM: 14% low-osmolar contrast (Iohexol), 86% iso-osmolar contrast (Iodixanol) Of the 3 modalities, the incidence of CIAKI was lowest with CT. "CIAKI was not independently associated with hospital admission or death."

C-81

Table C-68. CT-related adverse events, (continued)

Study	Study Design	Number of Patients	Diagnosis	Age, Years (Mean±SD)	% Male	N Harmed (%)	Adverse Events	Notes
Yang et al. 2008[143]	Prospective	67	NR	48±13	56.7	125 reports	Palpitation: 17 mild, 4 moderate, 1 severe Chest tightness: 12 mild, 2 moderate, 1 severe Dyspnea: 10 mild, 2 moderate, 1 severe Torridness: 64 mild Nausea/vomiting: 11 mild	Setting: hospital in Taiwan, Republic of China Timing: December 2005 to June 2006 CM: ionic iothalamate meglumine

CECT=Contrast-enhanced computed tomography; CIN=contrast-induced neuropathy; CPR=cardiopulmonary resuscitation; CTA=CT angiography; CTPA=CECT of the pulmonary arteries; NR=not reported; PE=pulmonary embolism; SCr=serum creatinine.

Table C-69. PET/CT-related adverse events

Study	Study Design	Number of Patients	Diagnosis	Age, Years (Mean±SD)	% Male	N Harmed (%)	Adverse Events	Notes
Codreanu et al. 2013[161]	Case report	1	Pyriform sinus cancer History of allergies	59	100	1 (100%)	Mild: 1 Recurring body rash and itching after injection of F18-FDG after 2 scans	Setting: NR Timing: NR Patient premedicated with Prednisone (50 mg) and Diphenhydramine (25 mg) when undergoing future scans.
Shah-Patel et al. 2009[140]	Retrospective chart review	106,800 total 3,359 PET/CT	NR	Range: 18–86	NR	5 (0.14)	Mild: 1 Itching or hives Severe: 4 Chest pain: 2 (1 before exam and 1 after FDG injection) Shortness of breath after IV injection: 2 (1 patient was premedicated for a known allergy to IV contrast)	Setting: Outpatient radiology in New York, NY Timing: over 4 years Total harms: 59 (0.06%) Patients requiring assistance from emergency medical services: 18 (31%)

CT=Computed tomography; F18-FDG=Fluorine-18-labeled fluorodeoxyglucose; IV=intravenous; mg=milligram; NR=not reported; NY=New York; PET=positron emission tomography; SD=standard deviation.

C-83

Table C-70. Physical and chemical characteristics of all currently marketed Gadolinium agents for MRI

Generic Name	Trade Name	Company	Acronym	Year Approved	Charge	Type	Dose (mml/kg)	Concentration (M)
Gadobenate dimeglumine	MultiHance®	Bracco Diagnostics, Princeton, NJ, USA	Gd-BOPTA	2004	Di-ionic	Liver-specific	0.1	0.5
Gadobutrol	Gadavist	Bayer HealthCare Pharmaceutical Inc., Wayne, NJ, USA	Gd-BT-DO3A	2011	Nonionic	ECF	0.1	1.0
Gadopentetate dimeglumine	Magnevist	Bayer HealthCare Pharmaceutical Inc., Wayne, NJ, USA	Gd-DTPA	1988	Di-ionic	ECF	0.1	0.5
Gadodiamide	Omniscan	GE Healthcare, Princeton, NJ, USA	Gd-DTPA-BMA	1993	Nonionic	ECF	0.1	0.5
Gadoversetamide	Optimark	Mallinckrodt, St. Louis, MO, USA	Gd-DTPA-BMEA	1999	Nonionic	ECF	0.1	0.5
Gadoxetic acid disodium salt	Eovist®	Bayer HealthCare, Wayne, NJ, USA	Gd-EOB-DTPA	2008	Di-ionic	Liver-specific	0.025	0.25
Gadoteridol	ProHance	Bracco Diagnostics, Princeton, NJ, USA	Gd-HP-DO3A	1992	Nonionic	ECF	0.1	0.5
Gadofosveset trisodium	Ablavar®	Lantheus Medical Imaging, North Billerica, MA, USA	MS325	2008	Tri-ionic	Blood-pool	0.03	0.25

ECF: Extracellular fluid.
Taken from Chang et al.[178] and Yang et al.[230]

Patterns of Care

Table C-71. Patterns of care for colorectal patients worldwide

Reference	Setting	Design	Non-invasive Imaging Methods Discussed	Findings
Melotti et al. 2013[213]	Italy	2,500 members of the Italian Society of Surgery were surveyed for preferred staging of distal rectal cancer. Overall response rate was 17.8% (444).	CT MRI PET/CT	**Staging single modalities:** T1 and T2: ERUS (preoperative and interim) T3 and T4: CT (preoperative and interim) Lymph node mesorectum: ERUS Lymph node extra-mesorectum: CT Metastases: CT **Staging combination modalities:** T1–T3: CT and ERUS (preoperative and interim) T4: CT and MRI (preoperative and interim) Lymph node mesorectum: ERUS and MRI Lymph node extra-mesorectum: CT and MRI Metastases: CT and FDG PET/CT

Table C-71. Patterns of care for colorectal patients worldwide, (continued)

Reference	Setting	Design	Non-invasive Imaging Methods Discussed	Findings
Bipat et al. 2012[223]	Netherlands Dutch hospitals (any type)	22 (64.7%) nuclear medicine physicists at hospitals with availability of PET/CT responded to a nuclear medicine survey 66 (75%) abdominal surgeons responded to a management survey 68 (77.3%) abdominal radiologists responded to a radiologist survey	CT MRI PET/CT	Management survey: For liver metastases, the first modality of choice was CT (78.8%) and US (18.2%). The second modality of choice was US (51.5%) and CT (16.7%). For lung metastases, chest CT or chest x-ray were dominantly used. For extrahepatic abdominal metastases, CT was dominantly used (n=55). Percent of hospitals "always using" imaging to detect liver metastases (97%), lung metastases (80.3%), and extrahepatic abdominal metastases (60.6%). Factors affecting choice of imaging modality (from most to least important) included evidence in the literature, availability, expertise, costs, personnel and waiting lists. Radiological survey: For detecting synchronous colorectal metastases, 68 radiologists reported using CT (98.5%), ultrasonography (45.6%), and MRI (22.7%). Nuclear medicine survey: For detecting synchronous colorectal metastases, 22 physicians (21 nuclear medicine) indicated PET/CT was solely performed in 14 (64%) hospitals. Practice patterns: While Dutch guidelines recommend either CT or MRI as a first choice for liver staging, use of MRI (and PET/CT) for staging was limited. These two modalities were predominately picked as a third choice for detecting lung and extrahepatic abdominal metastases.

Table C-71. Patterns of care for colorectal patients worldwide, (continued)

Reference	Setting	Design	Non-invasive Imaging Methods Discussed	Findings
Levine et al. 2012[219]	Royal Oak, MI, U.S.A. A multidisciplinary colorectal tumor clinic	Retrospective cohort study of 288 newly diagnosed colorectal patients. 248 patients were managed preoperatively outside the clinic while 40 patients were referred to the clinic.	Chest CT ERUS	Preoperative testing was completed in a significantly higher proportion of newly diagnosed colorectal clinic patients compared with nonclinic controls for abdominal CT (97.5% vs. 83.1%, p=0.03), chest CT (95% vs. 37.1%, p<0.0001) and ERUS for rectal cancer (88% vs. 37.7%, p<0.0001).
van der Geest et al. 2012[221]	Leiden region of the Netherlands 9 hospitals including university, hospital training surgical residents, and non-training	Population-based audit of Leiden Cancer Registry (2,211 stage I-III patients (1,667 colon, 544 rectal) surgically-treated from 2006 to 2008	MRI	A Chi-square test for time trends showed a statistically significant increase in use of preoperative MRI from 2006 to 2008 for rectal cancer patients, (73% to 85%; p=0.003) which remained after adjusting for case mix and hospital characteristics.
Habr-Gama et al. 2011[214]	Brazil	Web-based survey of 2,932 members of the Brazilian Society for Coloproctology, Brazilian College of Digestive Surgery, Brazilian College of Surgeons and Brazilian College of Medical Oncology for factors affecting management decisions in rectal cancer in clinical practice. Of 418 (14.2%) responders, 69.5% were surgeons and 30.5% were medical oncologists.	CT ERUS MRI	Preferred staging: MRI 63.6%, MRI 25.4%, ERUS 9.8%, other 1.2% Preferred staging by specialty: CT: 66.3% surgeons, 57.5% medical oncologists MRI or ERUS: 42.6% medical oncologists, 31.9% surgeons (p=0.03) Preferred preoperative staging: CT 55.2%, MRI or ERUS 43.1% Preferred interim staging: 66.9% CT, 32.1% MRI or ERUS Responders with >10 cases of rectal cancer/year "gave significantly more responses favoring MRI or ERUS for local staging."
Mroczkowski et al. 2011[215]	Poland Polish centers (number and type not specified)	Records of 709 rectal patients (67.6% stage III/IV) treated from 2008 to 2009.	CT ERUS MRI	Preoperatively, ERUS was performed in 23.7%, MRI in 2.5% and CT in 48.1%. "The accumulated results demonstrate definite shortcomings in diagnostic imaging performed prior to the surgery."

C-87

Table C-71. Patterns of care for colorectal patients worldwide, (continued)

Reference	Setting	Design	Non-invasive Imaging Methods Discussed	Findings
O'Grady et al. 2011[217]	U.S. Affiliate practices of Fox Chase Cancer Center Partners (based in OH, PA, and NJ)	Record review of 124 patients aged ≥65 diagnosed with stage III colon cancer between 2003 and 2006 to determine compliance with National Comprehensive Cancer Network guidelines	CT MRI	Compliance with documentation of initial workup and staging was high for chest imaging (100%), staging (98%), and CT abdomen/pelvis (93%).
Ooi et al. 2011[216]	Australia and New Zealand	174 members (specialist colorectal surgeons) of the Colorectal Surgical Society of Australia and New Zealand replied to a questionnaire on use of MRI for locally advanced rectal cancer patients. 108 (62.1%) responded, 98 (90.7%) completed. 81.5% practiced in Australia. 98% had access to MRI.	MRI	"93 (86.1%) surgeons would use MRI routinely as part of a work-up for suspected cT3 rectal cancer. The other 15 (13.9%) would use it selectively, particularly for tumors in the lower two-thirds of the rectum." 13.9% would use MRI in distal rectal cancer. "There is a move towards better patient selection with better preoperative imaging. Responses clearly demonstrate that variation exists despite the evidence-based guidelines and clinical practice."
Augestad et al. 2010[212]	28 countries in five continents (North American, Europe, Asia, South America, and Africa) University hospitals (78%), private (11.4%), city (9.8%), and rural (0.8%)	Survey of 173 colorectal surgeons from 173 international colorectal centers to identify regional differences in the preoperative management of rectal cancer. 123 (71%) responded.	CT ERUS MRI	For preoperative staging of rectal cancer, significantly more non-U.S. surgeons use MRI for all patients than U.S. surgeons (42.2% vs. 20.5%, p=0.03). Significantly more U.S. surgeons use ERUS for all patients than non-U.S. surgeons (43.6% vs. 21.1%, p=0.01). Similar rates for usage of CT in all patients was reported between U.S. and non-U.S. surgeons (56.4% vs. 53.5%, NS). Decision to use MRI for preoperative staging was significantly influenced by multidisciplinary team meetings (RR=3.62, 95% Confidence Interval 0.93 to 14.03; p=0.06).

Table C-71. Patterns of care for colorectal patients worldwide, (continued)

Reference	Setting	Design	Non-invasive Imaging Methods Discussed	Findings
McConnell et al. 2010[220]	Nova Scotia, Canada Urban/semi-urban community serviced by 1 tertiary hospital system and 1 community hospital	Prospective consecutive cohort study including 392 patients undergoing surgery for primary colorectal cancer from February 2002 to February 2004	CT MRI US	In multivariate analysis, rectal tumor (RR 4.4, p<0.001), community hospital (RR 1.9; p=0.04) and higher TNM staging (NS) were associated with undergoing preoperative imaging.
Cunningham et al. 2009[218]	New Zealand Public hospitals and private specialists	Population-based audit of New Zealand Cancer Registry; 642 individuals (308 Maori, 334 non-Maori) with histologically confirmed colon cancer	CT US	CT staging increased considerably from 1996 to 2003.
Lohsiriwat et al. 2009[211]	Thailand Secondary/tertiary hospitals (multidisciplinary teams and advanced facilities)	Survey of 50 board-certified colorectal surgeons (members of the Society of Colon and Rectal Surgeons Thailand) to assess current practice in rectal cancer surgery Of the 40 (80%) responders, 45% worked in a university hospital.	CT ERUS MRI US	Preoperative management: Routine use of CT/MRI of the pelvis: (90%), Routine use of ERUS: 7.5% for middle and low rectal cancer Preferred method of screening liver metastasis: CT: 67.5% US: 32.5% Due to limited availability of ERUS in Thailand, ERUS is seldom used in preoperative staging of rectal cancer.
Magne et al. 2009[210]	Belgium Academic and non-academic; public and private; Flemish and French speaking institutions	Surveyed specialists in GI radiotherapy at 16 hospitals regarding field of rectal cancer management (including staging) in order to reassess Belgian practice (comparing 2005 practices to 1999).	CT ERUS MRI	Most commonly used imaging for staging and restaging: contrast-enhanced CT The authors indicate use of CT "is sub-optimal since endorectal ultrasound or MRI are documented as being more accurate."

Table C-71. Patterns of care for colorectal patients worldwide, (continued)

Reference	Setting	Design	Non-invasive Imaging Methods Discussed	Findings
van Steenbergen et al. 2009[222]	Netherlands 10 community hospitals, 6 pathology departments, and 2 radio-therapy institutes	"To determine the extent of guideline implementation of the diagnostic approach in patients with CRC in southern Netherlands in 2005" the authors undertook a population-based audit of the Eindhoven Cancer Registry. 508 newly diagnosed colorectal (257 colon, 251 rectal) cancer patients	CT MRI	Preoperative staging with abdominal CT scan: 52% colon, 64% rectum Pelvic CT scan or MRI: 0% colon, 36% rectum

CRC=Colorectal cancer; CT=computed tomography; ERUS=endorectal ultrasonography; MRI=magnetic resonance imaging; NS=not significant; RR=relative risk; US=ultrasound.

Appendix D. Analyses and Risk of Bias Assessments

Preoperative Rectal T Staging

CT Versus ERUS

Table D-1. Pooled random effects meta-analysis: CT versus ERUS for preoperative primary rectal T staging

Measure	Correct	Understaged	Overstaged
Summary OR	0.359[a]	0.656	0.472
95% CI	0.238 to 0.541	0.438 to 0.894	0.28 to 0.798
I^2	67%	0%	50%
Favors	ERUS	ERUS	ERUS

[a] Odds ratio of getting an incorrect result

MRI Versus ERUS

Table D-2. Bivariate model MRI versus ERUS for preoperative primary rectal T staging

Test Characteristics	MRI	ERUS
Sensitivity (95% CI)	88.9% (79.0% to 94.4%)	88.0% (80.0% to 93.1%)
Specificity (95% CI)	85.3% (70.6% to 93.4%)	85.6% (65.8% to 94.9%)
Diagnostic OR (95% CI)	46.3 (17.8 to 120.4)	43.6 (11.6 to 164.5)
+ Likelihood ratio (95% CI)	6.1 (2.9 to 12.6)	6.1 (2.3 to 16.3)
- Likelihood ratio (95% CI)	0.13 (0.069 to 0.25)	0.14 (0.079 to 0.25)
Favors	No apparent difference	No apparent difference

Table D-3. Pooled random effects meta-analysis: MRI versus ERUS for preoperative primary rectal T staging

Measure	Correct	Understaged	Overstaged
Summary OR[a]	1.24	1.571	1.05
95% CI	0.835 to 1.84	0.605 to 4.083	0.518 to 2.16
I^2	24%	64%	42%
Favors	No statistically significant difference	No statistically significant difference	No statistically significant difference

[a] OR of getting an incorrect result

Figure D-1. HSROC of MRI for preoperative primary rectal T staging

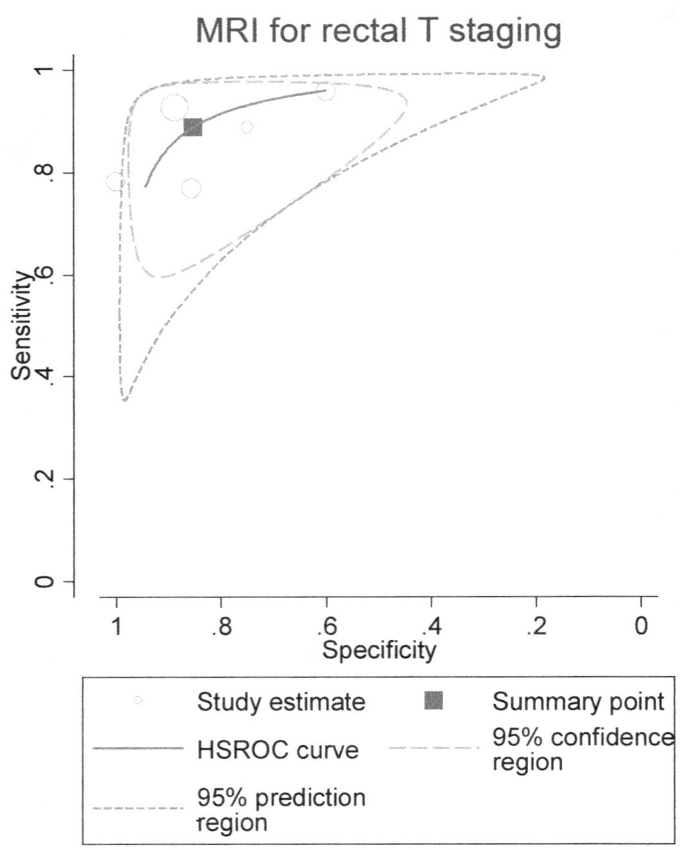

Figure D-2. HSROC of ERUS for preoperative primary rectal T staging

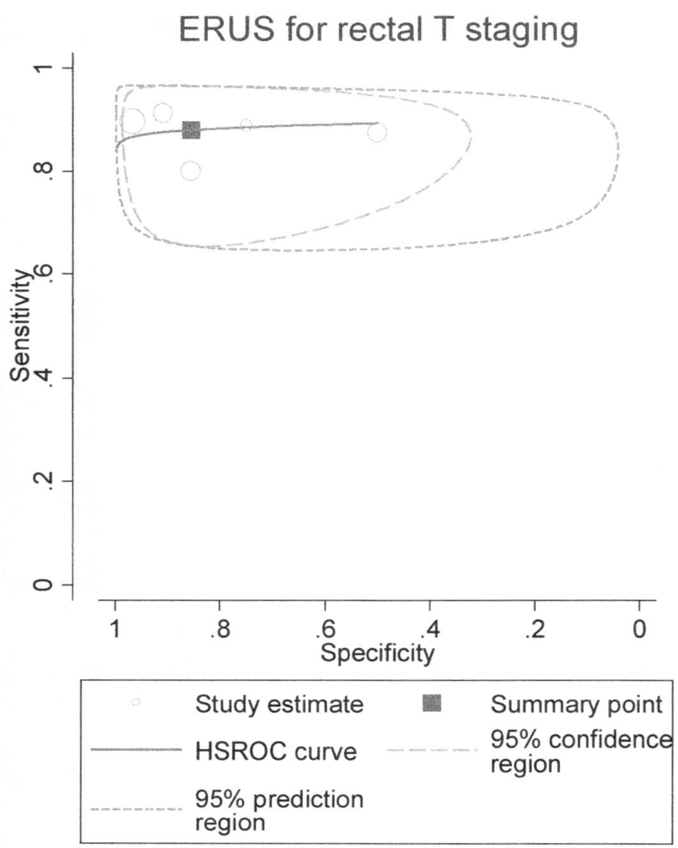

MRI Versus CT

Table D-4. Pooled random effects meta-analysis: MRI versus CT for preoperative rectal T staging

Measure	Correct	Understaged	Overstaged
Summary OR	0.317[a]	0.317	0.317
95% CI	0.056 to 1.784	0.027 to 3.646	0.028 to 3.653
I^2	0%	0%	0%
Favors	No statistically significant difference	No statistically significant difference	No statistically significant difference

[a] Odds ratio of an incorrect result

Preoperative Rectal N Staging

CT Versus ERUS

Table D-5. Bivariate model CT versus ERUS for preoperative primary rectal N staging

Test Characteristics	CT	ERUS
Sensitivity (95% CI)	39.6% (28.1% to 52.4%)	49.1% (34.9% to 63.5%)
Specificity (95% CI)	93.2% (58.8% to 99.2%)	71.7% (56.2% to 83.4%)
Diagnostic OR (95% CI)	9.0 (1.17 to 69.11)	2.45 (1.19 to 5.04)
+ Likelihood ratio (95% CI)	5.8 (0.82 to 41.5)	1.7 (1.1 to 2.8)
- Likelihood ratio (95% CI)	0.65 (0.54 to 0.77)	0.71 (0.53 to 0.94)
Favors	CT for specificity	ERUS for sensitivity

Figure D-3. HSROC of CT for preoperative primary rectal N staging

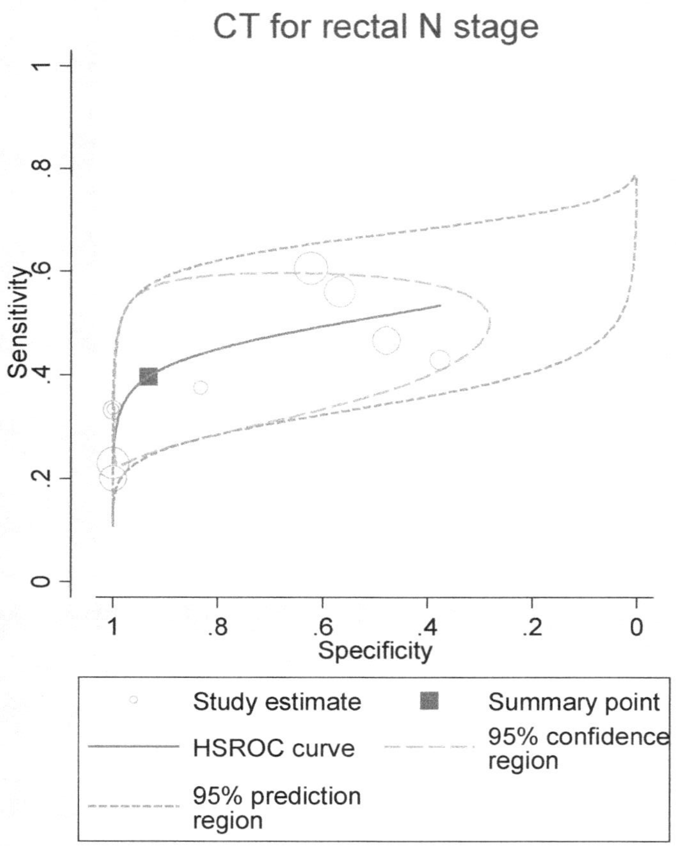

CT for rectal N stage

Figure D-4. HSROC of ERUS for preoperative primary rectal N staging

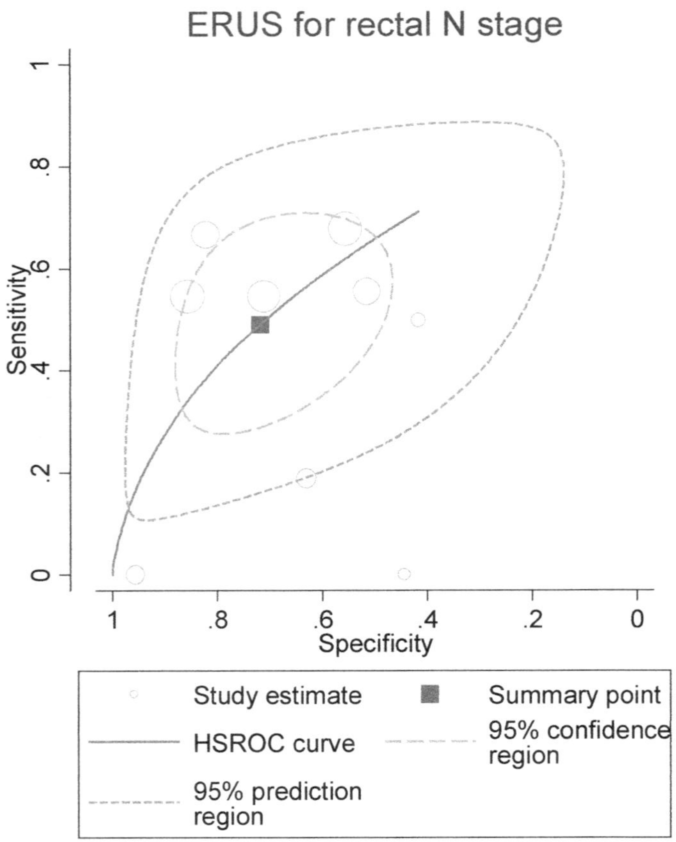

Table D-6. Pooled random effects meta-analysis: CT versus ERUS for preoperative primary rectal N staging

Measure	Correct	Understaged	Overstaged
Summary OR	1.13[a]	1.453	1.015
95% CI	0.85 to 1.503	0.854 to 2.473	0.571 to 1.801
I^2	29%	67%	57%
Favors	No statistically significant difference	No statistically significant difference	No statistically significant difference

[a] Odds ratio of getting an incorrect result

MRI Versus ERUS

Table D-7. Bivariate model MRI versus ERUS for preoperative primary rectal N staging

Test Characteristics	MRI	ERUS
Sensitivity (95% CI)	49.5% (36.0% to 63.1%)	63.7% (51.0% to 74.8%)
Specificity (95% CI)	69.7% (51.9% to 83.0%)	75.9% (46.1% to 92.1%)
Diagnostic OR (95% CI)	2.3 (0.73 to 6.9)	5.5 (1.5 to 19.9)
+ Likelihood ratio (95% CI)	1.6 (0.81 to 3.3)	2.6 (1.0 to 6.9)
- Likelihood ratio (95% CI)	0.72 (0.47 to 1.1)	0.48 (0.32 to 0.71)
Favors	ERUS	ERUS

Figure D-5. HSROC of MRI for preoperative primary rectal N staging

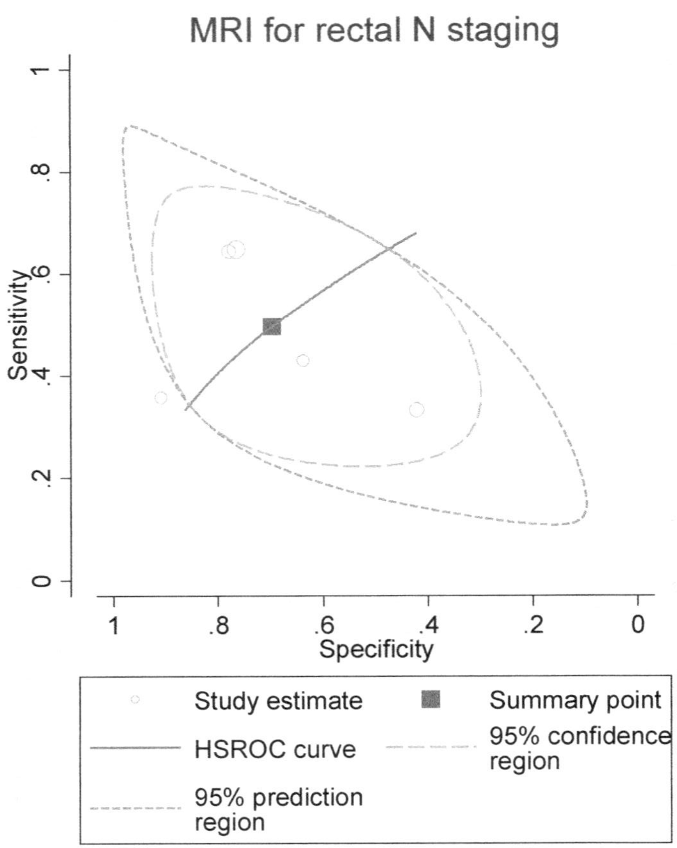

MRI for rectal N staging

Figure D-6. HSROC of ERUS for preoperative primary rectal N staging

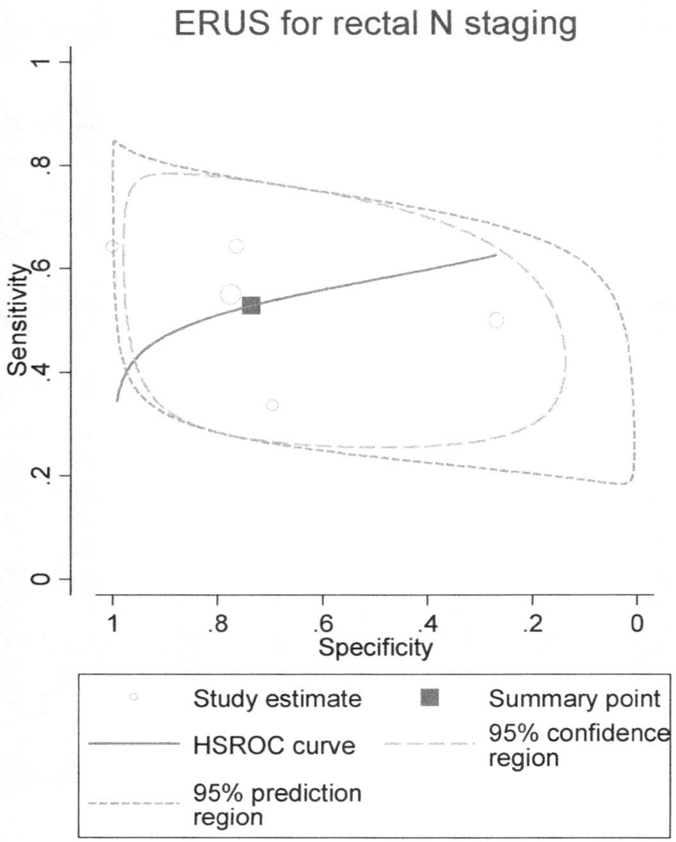

Table D-8. Pooled random effects meta-analysis: MRI versus ERUS for preoperative primary rectal N staging

Measure	Correct	Understaged	Overstaged
Summary odds ratio	0.882[a]	0.972	0.752
95% CI	0.542 to 1.408	0.563 to 1.679	0.457 to 1.237
I^2	51%	42%	14%
Favors	No statistically significant difference	No statistically significant difference	No statistically significant difference

[a] Odds ratio of getting an incorrect result

Change in Management

MRI Versus ERUS

Table D-9. Pooled random effects meta-analysis: MRI versus ERUS for preoperative primary rectal staging changes in management

Measure	Correct	Undertreated	Overtreated
Summary OR	0.326[a]	0.396	0.203
95% CI	0.052 to 2.045	0.129 to 1.216	0.011 to 3.847
I^2	95%	59%	85%
Favors	No statistically significant difference	No statistically significant difference	No statistically significant difference

[a] Odds ratio of getting an incorrect result

CT Versus MRI

Table D-10. Pooled random effects meta-analysis: CT versus MRI for preoperative rectal N staging

Measure	Correct	Understaged	Overstaged
Summary OR	1.023[a]	0.573	2.0
95% CI	0.465 to 2.245	0.338 to 0.973	1.233 to 3.229
I^2	73%	0%	0%
Favors	No statistically significant difference	CT	MRI

[a] OR of an incorrect result; OR < 1 indicates lower risk of error on CT; OR > 1 indicates higher risk of error on CT.

Preoperative Rectal M Staging

MRI Versus CT

Table D-11. Pooled random effects meta-analysis: MRI versus CT for preoperative colorectal M staging (per lesion)

Measure	Lesion Detection Rate
Summary OR[a]	1.334
95% CI	1.012 to 1.761
I^2	36%
Favors	MRI

[a] OR of detecting metastases

Rectal M Restaging

MRI Versus CT

Table D-12. Pooled random effects meta-analysis: MRI versus CT for interim colorectal M restaging (per lesion)

Measure	Lesion Detection Rate
Summary OR[a]	0.397
95% CI	0.111 to 1.418
I^2	85%
Favors	No statistically significant difference

[a] OR of getting an incorrect result

Colorectal M Staging

CT Versus PET/CT

Table D-13. Pooled data: CT versus PET/CT for preoperative colorectal M staging (per lesion)

Test Characteristics	CT	PET/CT
Sensitivity (95% CI)	83.6% (78.1% to 88.2%)	60.4% (53.7% to 66.9%)
I^2	0.0%	95.1%
Specificity (95% CI)	Not calculated	Not calculated
Favors	Insufficient	Insufficient

Interim Rectal T Restaging

MRI Versus CT Versus ERUS

Table D-14. Pooled random effects meta-analysis: MRI versus CT versus ERUS for interim rectal T restaging

Measure	Accuracy MRI Versus CT	Accuracy MRI Versus ERUS	Accuracy CT Versus ERUS
Summary OR[a]	0.943	0.948	0.907
95% CI	0.652 to 1.34	0.471 to 1.907	0.41 to 2.011
I^2	0%	67%	74%
Favors	No statistically significant difference	No statistically significant difference	No statistically significant difference

[a] Odds ratio of getting an inaccurate result

Interim Rectal N Restaging

MRI Versus CT Versus ERUS

Table D-15. Pooled random effects meta-analysis: MRI versus CT versus ERUS for interim rectal N restaging

Measure	Accuracy MRI Versus CT	Accuracy MRI Versus ERUS	Accuracy CT Versus ERUS
Summary OR[a]	0.874	1.457	1.531
95% CI	0.609 to 1.253	0.487 to 4.362	0.727 to 3.224
I^2	0%	86%	70%
Favors	No statistically significant difference	No statistically significant difference	No statistically significant difference

[a] Odds ratio of getting an inaccurate result

Publication Bias

Figure D-7. Funnel plot of CT versus ERUS, accuracy of rectal T staging

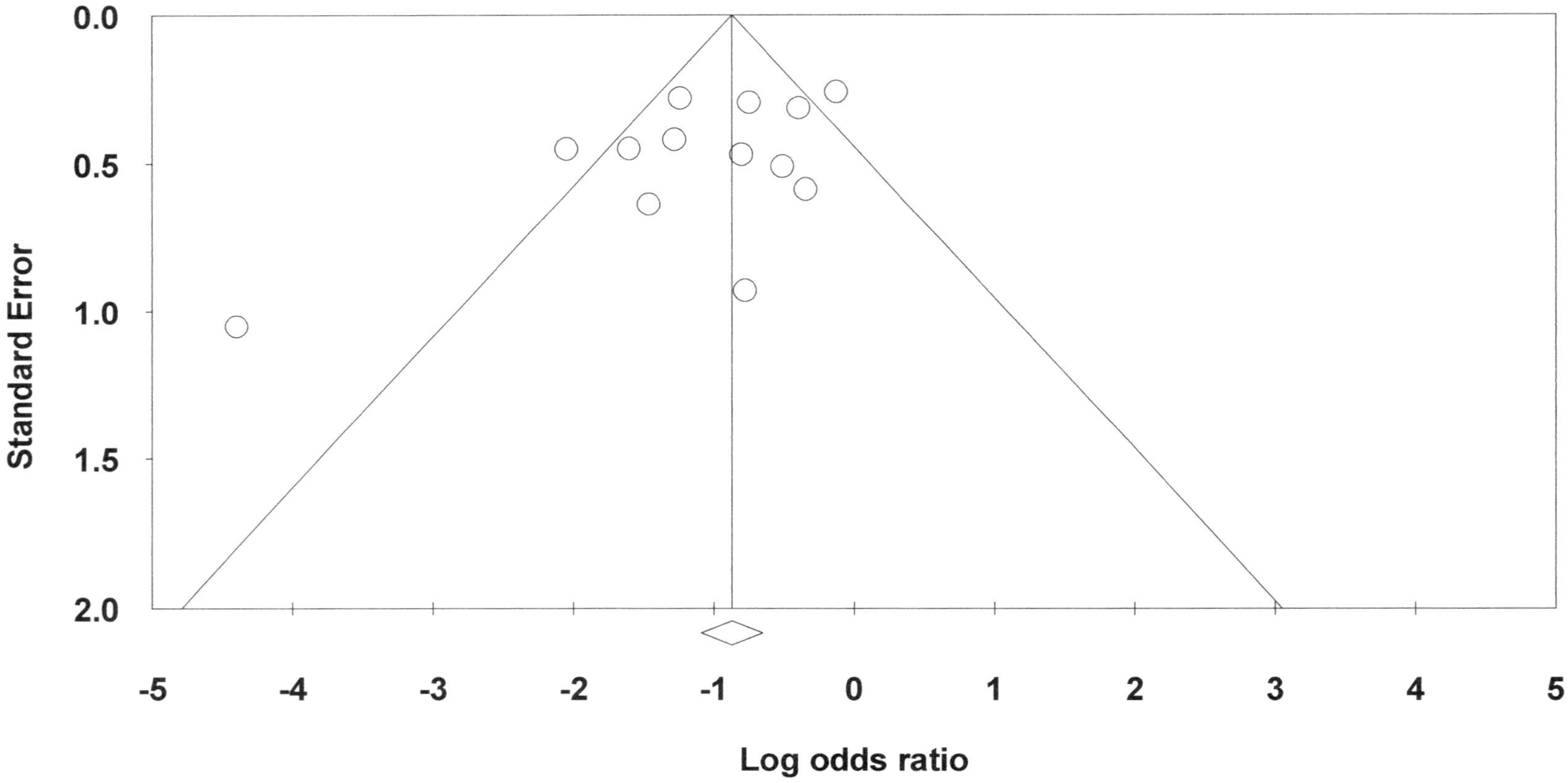

Figure D-8. Effect size by publication date, CT versus ERUS, accuracy of rectal T staging

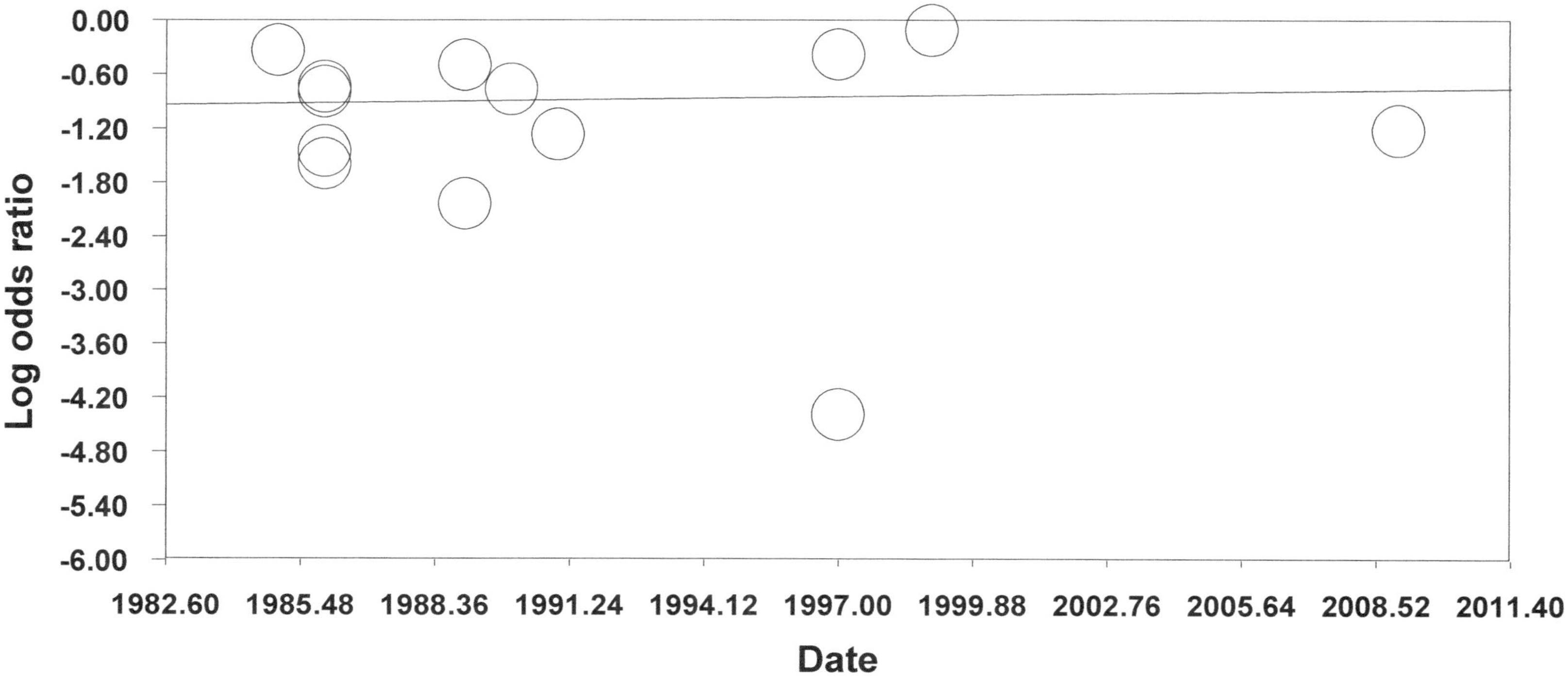

Figure D-9. Funnel plot of MRI versus ERUS, accuracy of rectal T staging

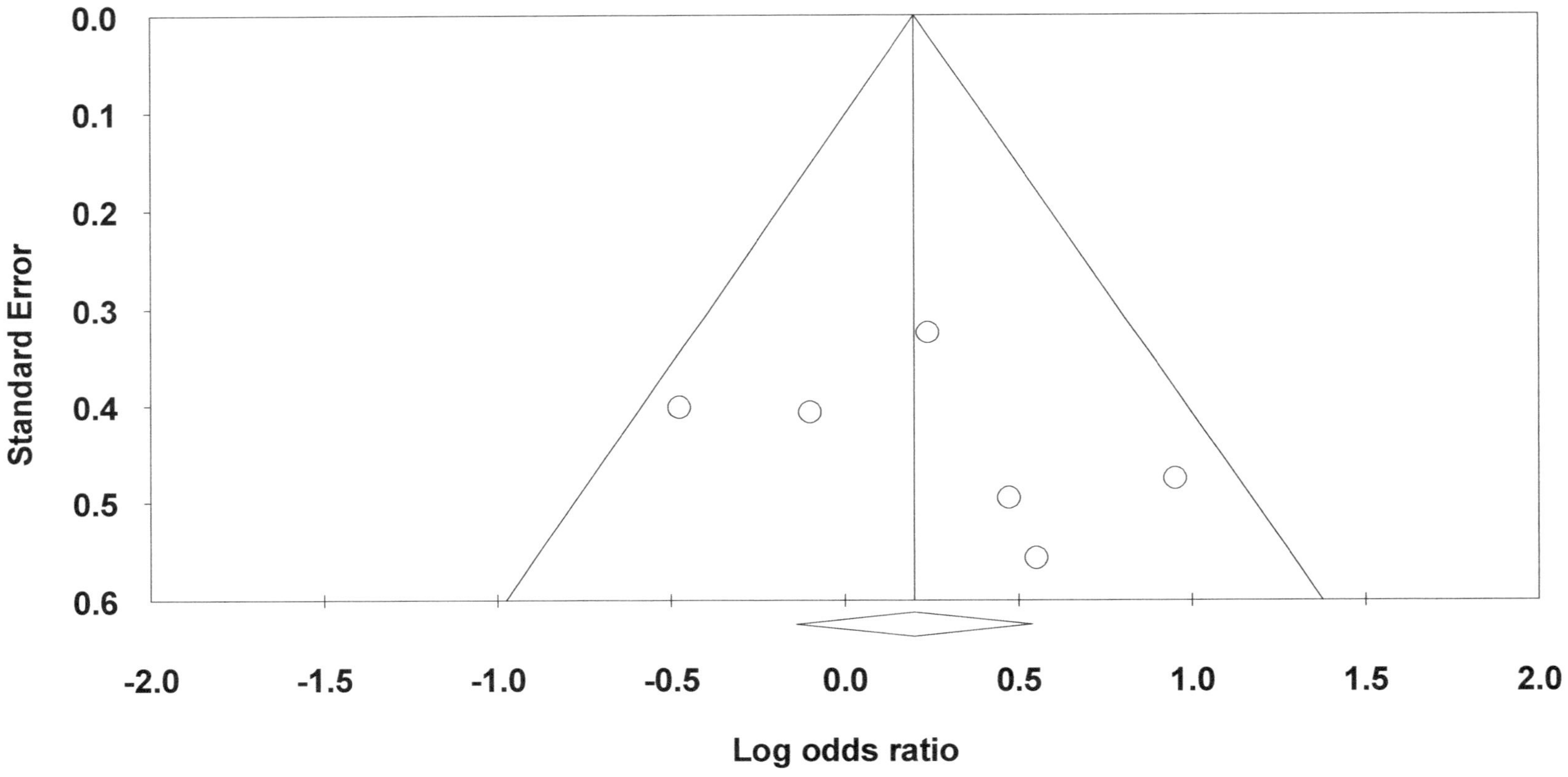

Figure D-10. Effect size by publication date, MRI versus ERUS, accuracy of rectal T staging

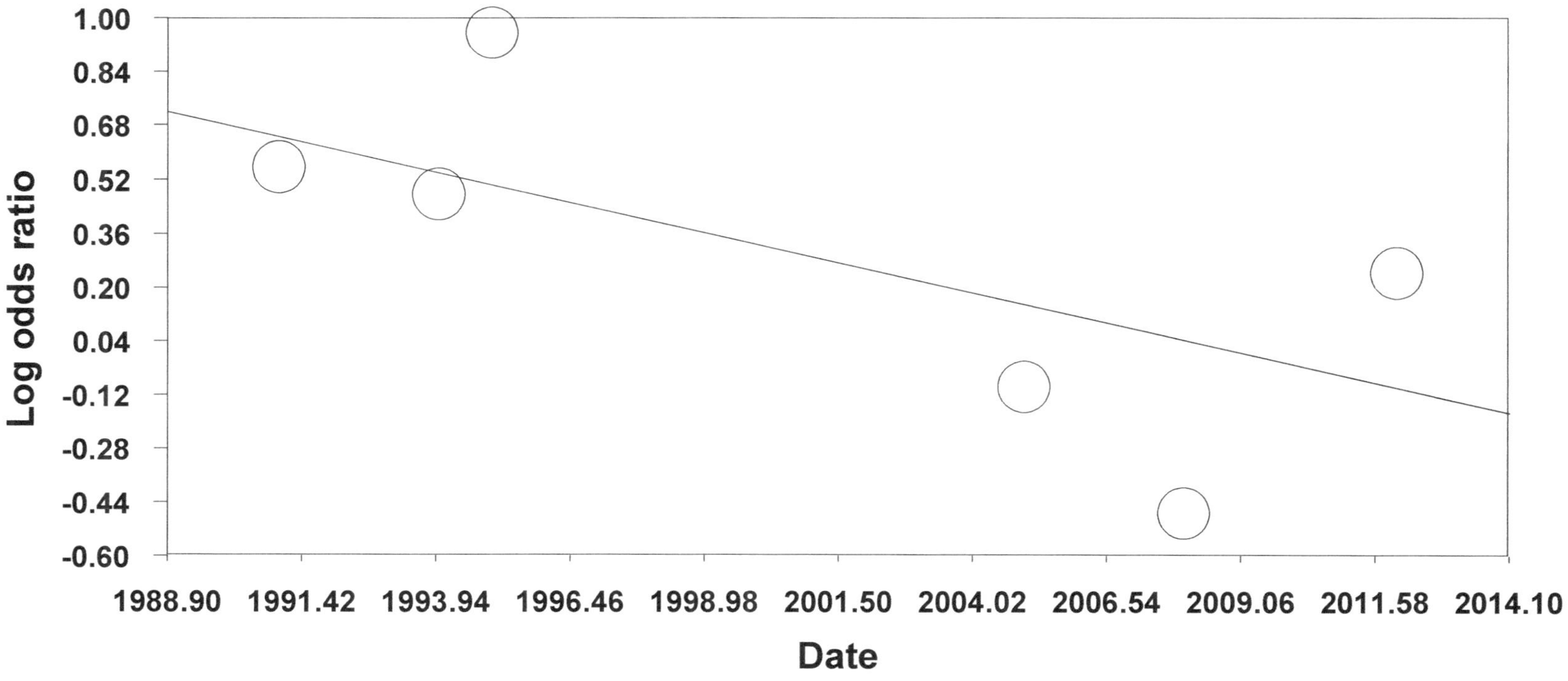

Sensitivity Analyses on External Correlations

Table D-16. Sensitivity analyses using different test-test correlations

Timing	Rectal or Colorectal	Type of Staging	Comparison	Primary Analysis using correlation=0.5 (Summary OR and 95% Confidence Interval)	Sensitivity Analysis using correlation=0.1 (Summary OR and 95% Confidence Interval)	Sensitivity Analysis using correlation=0.9 (Summary OR and 95% Confidence Interval)	Important Change Upon Sensitivity Analysis?	Nature of the Change
Pretreatment	Rectal	T stage	MRI vs. ERUS	1.24 (0.835 to 1.84)	1.22 (0.78 to 1.93)	1.30 (0.89 to 1.89)	No	NA
Pretreatment	Rectal	T stage	MRI vs. ERUS	1.571 (0.605 to 4.083)	1.605 (0.605 to 4.255)	1.342 (0.477 to 3.774)	No	NA
Pretreatment	Rectal	T stage	MRI vs. ERUS	1.05 (0.518 to 2.16)	0.992 (0.498 to 1.976)	1.149 (0.481 to 2.747)	No	NA
Pretreatment	Rectal	T stage	ERUS vs. CT	0.359 (0.238 to 0.541)	0.376 (0.250 to 0.566)	0.322 (0.215 to 0.482)	No	NA
Pretreatment	Rectal	T stage	ERUS vs. CT	0.626 (0.438 to 0.894)	0.619 (0.386 to 0.993)	0.621 (0.451 to 0.855)	No	NA
Pretreatment	Rectal	T stage	ERUS vs. CT	0.472 (0.28 to 0.798)	0.487 (0.29 to 0.817)	0.465 (0.292 to 0.739)	No	NA
Pretreatment	Rectal	T stage	MRI vs. CT	0.317 (0.056 to 1.784)	0.317 (0.035 to 2.867)	0.317 (0.11 to 0.914)	Yes	Became statistically significant if a correlation of 0.9 was used
Pretreatment	Rectal	T stage	MRI vs. CT	0.317 (0.027 to 3.646)	0.317 (0.014 to 7.139)	0.317 (0.071 to 1.413)	No	NA
Pretreatment	Rectal	T stage	MRI vs. CT	0.318 (0.028 to 3.653)	0.318 (0.014 to 7.135)	0.318 (0.071 to 1.421)	No	NA
Pretreatment	Rectal	N stage	MRI vs. ERUS	0.882 (0.542 to 1.408)	0.853 (0.537 to 1.357)	0.915 (0.584 to 1.435)	No	NA
Pretreatment	Rectal	N stage	MRI vs. ERUS	0.972 (0.563 to 1.679)	1.011 (0.591 to 1.727)	0.932 (0.557 to 1.561)	No	NA
Pretreatment	Rectal	N stage	MRI vs. ERUS	0.752 (0.457 to 1.237)	0.743 (0.409 to 1.349)	0.809 (0.504 to 1.296)	No	NA
Pretreatment	Rectal	N stage	ERUS vs. CT	1.13 (0.85 to 1.503)	1.11 (0.826 to 1.504)	1.2 (0.923 to 1.548)	No	NA

Table D-16. Sensitivity analyses using different test-test correlations, (continued)

Timing	Rectal or Colorectal	Type of Staging	Comparison	Primary Analysis using correlation=0.5 (Summary OR and 95% Confidence Interval)	Sensitivity Analysis using correlation=0.1 (Summary OR and 95% Confidence Interval)	Sensitivity Analysis using correlation=0.9 (Summary OR and 95% Confidence Interval)	Important Change Upon Sensitivity Analysis?	Nature of the Change
Pretreatment	Rectal	N stage	ERUS vs. CT	1.453 (0.854 to 2.473)	1.369 (0.803 to 2.332)	1.561 (0.959 to 2.542)	No	NA
Pretreatment	Rectal	N stage	ERUS vs. CT	1.015 (0.571 to 1.801)	1.013 (0.548 to 1.872)	1.092 (0.718 to 1.66)	No	NA
Pretreatment Accuracy	Rectal	N stage	MRI vs. CT	1.316 (0.709 to 2.243)	1.379 (0.752 to 2.529)	1.256 (0.680 to 2.322)	No	NA
Pretreatment Understaging	Rectal	N stage	MRI vs. CT	1.743 (1.028 to 2.957)	1.743 (0.859 to 1.538)	1.585 (0.958 to 2.625)	Yes	Became non-statistically significant if either correlation of 0.1 or 0.9 were used or if Hodgman study removed (0.15T magnet)
Pretreatment Overstaging	Rectal	N stage	MRI vs. CT	0.498 (0.308 to 0.806)	0.498 (0.262 to 0.947)	0.499 (0.399 to 0.625)	No	NA
Pretreatment	Colorectal	Detection of metastases	MRI vs. CT	1.334 (1.012 to 1.761)	1.349 (1.023 to 1.778)	1.331 (1.012 to 1.749)	No	NA
Restaging	Rectal	T stage	CT vs. MRI	0.943 (0.652 to 1.34)	0.934 (0.576 to 1.516)	0.934 (0.795 to 1.098)	No	NA
Restaging	Rectal	T stage	CT vs. ERUS	0.907 (0.410 to 2.011)	0.879 (0.400 to 1.931)	0.937 (0.421 to 2.085)	No	NA
Restaging	Rectal	T stage	MRI vs. ERUS	0.948 (0.471 to 1.907)	0.914 (0.460 to 1.817)	0.983 (0.486 to 1.988)	No	NA
Restaging	Rectal	N stage	MRI vs. CT	0.874 (0.609 to 1.253)	0.874 (0.538 to 1.418)	0.919 (0.651 to 1.298)	No	NA
Restaging	Rectal	N stage	CT vs. ERUS	1.531 (0.727 to 3.224)	1.469 (0.709 to 3.045)	1.596 (0.753 to 3.384)	No	NA
Restaging	Rectal	N stage	MRI vs. ERUS	1.457 (0.487 to 4.362)	1.418 (0.476 to 4.225)	1.497 (0.499 to 4.493)	No	NA

Table D-16. Sensitivity analyses using different test-test correlations, (continued)

Timing	Rectal or Colorectal	Type of Staging	Comparison	Primary Analysis using correlation=0.5 (Summary OR and 95% Confidence Interval)	Sensitivity Analysis using correlation=0.1 (Summary OR and 95% Confidence Interval)	Sensitivity Analysis using correlation=0.9 (Summary OR and 95% Confidence Interval)	Important Change Upon Sensitivity Analysis?	Nature of the Change
Restaging	Colorectal	Detection of metastases	CT vs. MRI	0.397 (0.111 to 1.418)	0.402 (0.104 to 1.551)	0.409 (0.157 to 1.062)	No	NA
Treatment selection	Rectal	Correct treatment	MRI vs. ERUS	0.326 (0.052 to 2.045)	0.324 (0.052 to 2.032)	0.329 (0.052 to 2.058)	No	NA
Treatment selection	Rectal	Correct treatment	MRI vs. ERUS	0.396 (0.129 to 1.216)	0.341 (0.128 to 0.91)	0.46 (0.142 to 1.489)	Yes, but no change to conclusion	Became statistically significant if a correlation of 0.1 was used
Treatment selection	Rectal	Correct treatment	MRI vs. ERUS	0.203 (0.011 to 3.847)	0.196 (0.01 to 3.721)	0.21 (0.11 to 3.97)	No	NA

ERUS=endorectal ultrasound; MRI=magnetic resonance imaging; NR=not reported; pT=pathologic tumor stage; T=tumor stage.

Risk of Bias of Individual Studies

ECRI Instrument for Controlled/Comparative Studies

1. Were patients randomly assigned to the study's groups?
2. Did the study use appropriate randomization methods?
3. Was there concealment of group allocation?
4. For nonrandomized trials, did the study employ any other methods to enhance group comparability?
5. Was the process of assigning patients to groups made independently from physician and patient preference?
6. Did the patients in different study groups have similar levels of performance on the outcome of interest at the time they were assigned to groups?
7. Were the study groups comparable for all other important factors at the time they were assigned to groups?
8. Did the study enroll all suitable patients or consecutive suitable patients?
9. Was the comparison of interest prospectively planned?
10. If the patients received ancillary treatment(s), was there a ≤5 percent difference between groups in the proportion of patients receiving each specific ancillary treatment?
11. Were the two groups treated concurrently?
12. Was compliance with treatment ≥85 percent in both of the study's groups?
13. Were patients blinded to the treatment they received?
14. Was the healthcare provider blinded to the groups to which the patients were assigned?
15. Were those who assessed the patient's outcomes blinded to the group to which the patients were assigned?
16. Was the integrity of blinding of patients, physicians, or outcome assessors tested and found to be preserved?
17. Was the outcome measure of interest objective and was it objectively measured?
18. Was a standard instrument used to measure the outcome?
19. Was there ≤15 percent difference in the length of followup for the two groups?
20. Did ≥85 percent of the patients complete the study?
21. Was there a ≤15 percent difference in completion rates in the study's groups?
22. Was the funding for this study derived from a source that would not benefit financially from results in a particular direction?

Table D-17. Risk of bias of individual studies with two or more groups

Study	1. RCT?	2. Appropriate RCT?	3. Concealment?	4. Group comparability?	5. Group assignment?	6. Groups similar on outcome?	7. Groups similar?	8. All/consecutive enrollment?	9. Prospective?	10. Ancillary treatments?	11. Concurrent?	12. Compliance?	13. Patients blinded?	14. Provider blinded?	15. Assessor blinded?	16. Blinding tested?	17. Objective?	18. Standard?	19. Followup?	20. Completion?	21. Attrition?	22. Funding?	Risk of Bias
Yimei et al. 2012[93]	No	No	No	No	No	NR	Yes	Yes	No	Yes	Yes	Yes	No	No	No	No	No	Yes	Yes	Yes	Yes	Yes	Moderate
Mo et al. 2002[165]	No	No	No	No	NR	No	No	Yes	Yes	Yes	Yes	Yes	No	No	NR	NR	No	Yes	Yes	Yes	Yes	NR	High
Lupo et al. 1996[190]	No	No	No	No	NR	Yes	Yes	NR	NR	Yes	Yes	Yes	No	No	Yes	No	No	Yes	Yes	Yes	Yes	NR	Moderate

Instrument for Single-Group Diagnostic Test Performance Studies

1. Did the study enroll all, consecutive, or a random sample of patients?
2. Were more than 85 percent of the approached/eligible patients enrolled?
3. Were the patient inclusion and exclusion criteria applied consistently to all patients?
4. Was the study affected by obvious spectrum bias?
5. Did the study account for inter-reader differences?
6. Were readers of the diagnostic test of interest blinded to the results of the reference standard?
7. Were readers of the reference standard blinded to the results of the diagnostic test of interest?
8. Were readers of the diagnostic test of interest blinded to all other clinical information?
9. Were readers of the reference standard blinded to all other clinical information?
10. Were patients assessed by a reference standard regardless of the test's results?
11. Were all patients assessed by the same reference standard regardless of the test's results?
12. If the study reported data for a single diagnostic threshold, was the threshold chosen *a priori*?
13. Were the study results unaffected by intervening treatments or disease progression/regression?
14. Were at least 85 percent of the enrolled patients accounted for?
15. Was the funding for the study derived from a source that does not have a financial interest in its results?

Table D-18. Risk of bias of individual studies: single-group studies

Study	1. All/consecutive enrollment?	2. 85% enrolled?	3. Consistent inclusion?	4. No spectrum bias?	5. Inter-reader difference?	6. Reader blinded standard?	7. Reader standard blinded test?	8. Reader blinded clinical?	9. Reader standard blinded clinical?	10. All standard?	11. Same standard?	12. Threshold?	13. Intervening treatment?	14. Attrition?	15. Funding?	Risk of Bias
Halefoglu et al. 2008[94]	Yes	Yes	Yes	Yes	No	Yes	NR	Yes	NR	Yes	Yes	Yes	Yes	Yes	NR	Low
Rafaelsen et al. 2008[188]	Yes	Yes	Yes	Yes	Yes	No	NR	NR	NR	Yes	Yes	Yes	Yes	Yes	NR	Moderate
Bianchi et al. 2005[95]	Yes	Yes	Yes	No	No	Yes	NR	NR	NR	Yes	Yes	Yes	Yes	Yes	NR	Moderate
Brown et al. 2004[125]	Yes	NR	Yes	No	No	NR	NR	NR	NR	Yes	No	Yes	No	Yes	Yes	Moderate
Starck et al. 1995[96]	Yes	NR	NR	Yes	No	Yes	Yes	Yes	Yes	Yes	Yes	Yes	NR	Yes	NR	Moderate
Thaler et al. 1994[97]	Yes	Yes	Yes	Yes	No	Yes	No	NR	NR	Yes	Yes	Yes	Yes	Yes	NR	Low
Waizer et al. 1991[98]	NR	NR	Yes	No	NR	NR	NR	NR	NR	Yes	Yes	Yes	Yes	Yes	NR	Moderate
Berger-Kulemann et al. 2012[200]	Yes	Yes	Yes	No	Yes	Yes	Yes	NR	NR	Yes	Yes	Yes	Yes	Yes	NR	Low
Kulemann et al. 2011[201]	Yes	Yes	Yes	No	NR	Yes	Yes	NR	NR	Yes	Yes	Yes	No	Yes	NR	Moderate
van Kessel et al. 2011[202]	No	NR	NR	Yes	Yes	Yes	No	NR	No	Yes	No	Yes	NR	Yes	NR	Moderate
Taylor et al. 2007[119]	Yes	Yes	Yes	No	No	Yes	Yes	NR	NR	Yes	Yes	Yes	Yes	Yes	NR	Moderate
Arii et al. 2006[117]	Yes	Yes	Yes	Yes	Yes	No	NR	NR	NR	Yes	No	Yes	NR	Yes	Yes	Moderate
Bartolozzi et al. 2004[120]	Yes	NR	Yes	Yes	Yes	Yes	Yes	Yes	Yes	Yes	Yes	Yes	NR	Yes	NR	Low

Table D-18. Risk of bias of individual studies: single-group studies (continued)

Study	1. All/consecutive enrollment?	2. 85% enrolled?	3. Consistent inclusion?	4. No spectrum bias?	5. Inter-reader difference?	6. Reader blinded standard?	7. Reader standard blinded test?	8. Reader blinded clinical?	9. Reader standard blinded clinical?	10. All standard?	11. Same standard?	12. Threshold?	13. Intervening treatment?	14. Attrition?	15. Funding?	Risk of Bias
Bhattacharjya et al. 2004[121]	Yes	Yes	Yes	Yes	No	NR	Yes	Yes	NR	Yes	No	Yes	No	Yes	NR	Moderate
Bohm et al. 2004[122]	Yes	NR	Yes	No	NR	NR	NR	NR	NR	Yes	No	Yes	NR	Yes	NR	Moderate
Matsuoka et al. 2003[112]	NR	NR	NR	Yes	NR	NR	NR	Yes	NR	Yes	Yes	Yes	No	Yes	NR	Moderate
Blomqvist et al. 2002[115]	Yes	NR	NR	No	Yes	Yes	NR	No	NR	Yes	Yes	Yes	No	Yes	Yes	Moderate
Lencioni et al. 1998[123]	Yes	Yes	Yes	Yes	NR	Yes	NR	Yes	NR	Yes	Yes	Yes	Yes	Yes	NR	Low
Strotzer et al. 1997[124]	Yes	Yes	Yes	No	Yes	Yes	NR	NR	NR	Yes	Yes	Yes	NR	Yes	NR	Low
Guinet et al. 1990[113]	NR	NR	Yes	No	No	Yes	NR	Yes	NR	Yes	Yes	Yes	NR	Yes	NR	Moderate
Hodgman et al. 1986[114]	No	NR	Yes	No	NR	Yes	No	NR	NR	Yes	Yes	Yes	Yes	Yes	NR	Moderate
Wickramasinghe and Samarasekera 2012[126]	Yes	Yes	Yes	Yes	No	NR	NR	NR	NR	Yes	Yes	Yes	Yes	Yes	NR	Low
Ju et al. 2009[99]	NR	NR	NR	Yes	NR	Yes	NR	NR	NR	Yes	Yes	Yes	Yes	Yes	NR	Moderate
Huh et al. 2008[164]	Yes	Yes	Yes	Yes	Yes	Yes	Yes	NR	NR	Yes	Yes	Yes	Yes	Yes	NR	Low
Harewood et al. 2002[127]	Yes	NR	Yes	Yes	No	Yes	No	NR	NR	Yes	Yes	Yes	No	Yes	NR	Moderate
Kim et al. 1999[100]	Yes	Yes	Yes	Yes	NR	NR	NR	NR	NR	Yes	Yes	Yes	Yes	Yes	NR	Moderate
Osti et al. 1997[101]	NR	NR	NR	Yes	NR	NR	NR	NR	NR	Yes	Yes	Yes	Yes	Yes	NR	Moderate

D-25

Table D-18. Risk of bias of individual studies: single-group studies (continued)

Study	1. All/consecutive enrollment?	2. 85% enrolled?	3. Consistent inclusion?	4. No spectrum bias?	5. Inter-reader difference?	6. Reader blinded standard?	7. Reader standard blinded test?	8. Reader blinded clinical?	9. Reader standard blinded clinical?	10. All standard?	11. Same standard?	12. Threshold?	13. Intervening treatment?	14. Attrition?	15. Funding?	Risk of Bias
Ramana et al. 1997[102]	NR	NR	NR	Yes	NR	NR	NR	NR	NR	Yes	Yes	Yes	Yes	Yes	NR	Moderate
Fleshman et al. 1992[116]	NR	NR	Yes	Yes	NR	NR	NR	NR	NR	Yes	Yes	Yes	No	Yes	NR	Moderate
Milsom et al. 1992[118]	Yes	Yes	Yes	Yes	NR	NR	NR	NR	NR	Yes	Yes	Yes	Yes	Yes	NR	Moderate
Goldman et al. 1991[103]	NR	NR	NR	Yes	No	Yes	Yes	NR	NR	Yes	Yes	Yes	Yes	Yes	NR	Moderate
Pappalardo et al. 1990[104]	Yes	Yes	Yes	Yes	NR	NR	NR	NR	NR	Yes	Yes	Yes	Yes	Yes	NR	Moderate
Rotte et al. 1989[105]	NR	NR	NR	Yes	NR	NR	NR	NR	NR	Yes	Yes	Yes	Yes	Yes	NR	Moderate
Waizer et al. 1989[106]	NR	NR	NR	Yes	No	NR	NR	NR	NR	Yes	Yes	Yes	Yes	Yes	NR	Moderate
Beynon et al. 1986[107]	NR	NR	NR	Yes	No	NR	No	NR	NR	Yes	Yes	Yes	Yes	Yes	NR	Moderate
Kramann and Hildebrandt 1986[108]	NR	NR	NR	Yes	NR	Yes	Yes	NR	NR	Yes	Yes	Yes	Yes	Yes	Yes	Moderate
Rifkin and Wechsler 1986[109]	NR	NR	NR	Yes	NR	Yes	Yes	NR	NR	Yes	Yes	Yes	Yes	Yes	NR	Moderate
Rifkin and Marks 1986[110]	NR	Yes	Yes	Yes	NR	NR	NR	NR	NR	Yes	Yes	Yes	Yes	Yes	NR	Moderate
Romano et al. 1985[111]	NR	NR	NR	Yes	No	Yes	Yes	NR	NR	Yes	Yes	Yes	Yes	Yes	NR	Moderate
Engledow et al. 2012[128]	Yes	Yes	Yes	Yes	No	NR	No	NR	NR	No	No	Yes	Yes	Yes	Yes	Moderate
Uchiyama et al. 2012[89]	Yes	NR	NR	No	No	NR	No	NR	NR	Yes	Yes	Yes	NR	Yes	NR	Moderate

Table D-18. Risk of bias of individual studies: single-group studies (continued)

Study	1. All/consecutive enrollment?	2. 85% enrolled?	3. Consistent inclusion?	4. No spectrum bias?	5. Inter-reader difference?	6. Reader blinded standard?	7. Reader standard blinded test?	8. Reader blinded clinical?	9. Reader standard blinded clinical?	10. All standard?	11. Same standard?	12. Threshold?	13. Intervening treatment?	14. Attrition?	15. Funding?	Risk of Bias
Ramos et al. 2011[19]	Yes	Yes	Yes	Yes	No	Yes	NR	NR	No	Yes	No	Yes	NR	Yes	Yes	Moderate
Orlacchio et al. 2009[90]	Yes	NR	NR	NR	No	Yes	NR	NR	NR	Yes	No	Yes	NR	Yes	NR	Moderate
Lubezky et al. 2007[91]	Yes	Yes	NR	Yes	Yes	NR	NR	NR	NR	Yes	No	Yes	No	Yes	NR	Moderate
Kim et al. 2011[88]	Yes	NR	NR	NR	No	NR	NR	NR	NR	Yes	NR	Yes	Yes	Yes	Yes	Moderate
Martellucci et al. 2012[199]	Yes	Yes	Yes	Yes	No	Yes	NR	NR	NR	Yes	Yes	Yes	No	Yes	NR	Moderate
Pomerri et al. 2011[163]	Yes	NR	Yes	Yes	Yes	NR	NR	NR	NR	Yes	Yes	Yes	No	Yes	Yes	Low
Barbaro et al. 1995[92]	NR	NR	NR	No	NR	No	NR	NR	NR	Yes	Yes	Yes	NR	Yes	NR	Moderate
Kim et al. 2004[186]	Yes	Yes	Yes	Yes	Yes	No	Yes	No	NR	Yes	Yes	Yes	Yes	Yes	NR	Moderate
Hunerbein et al. 2000[187]	Yes	No	Yes	Yes	No	No	NR	NR	NR	Yes	Yes	Yes	No	Yes	NR	Moderate
Wicherts et al. 2011[191]	Yes	No	Yes	Yes	Yes	Yes	No	NR	NR	Yes	Yes	Yes	No	Yes	NR	Moderate
Skriver et al. 1992[189]	NR	NR	NR	Yes	NR	Yes	Yes	NR	NR	Yes	Yes	Yes	Yes	Yes	NR	Moderate
Koh et al. 2012[192]	Yes	Yes	Yes	Yes	Yes	Yes	No	NR	NR	Yes	No	Yes	No	Yes	Yes	Low
Lambregts et al. 2011[203]	Yes	No	Yes	Yes	Yes	Yes	NR	NR	NR	Yes	Yes	Yes	No	Yes	NR	Moderate
Jao et al. 2010[193]	Yes	Yes	Yes	Yes	Yes	Yes	NR	NR	NR	Yes	Yes	Yes	Yes	Yes	NR	Low
Kim et al. 2010[229]	Yes	Yes	Yes	Yes	Yes	Yes	Yes	NR	NR	Yes	Yes	Yes	Yes	Yes	Yes	Low

Table D-18. Risk of bias of individual studies: single-group studies (continued)

Study	1. All/consecutive enrollment?	2. 85% enrolled?	3. Consistent inclusion?	4. No spectrum bias?	5. Inter-reader difference?	6. Reader blinded standard?	7. Reader standard blinded test?	8. Reader blinded clinical?	9. Reader standard blinded clinical?	10. All standard?	11. Same standard?	12. Threshold?	13. Intervening treatment?	14. Attrition?	15. Funding?	Risk of Bias
Futterer et al. 2008[197]	Yes	Yes	Yes	Yes	Yes	No	Yes	NR	NR	Yes	Yes	Yes	Yes	Yes	NR	Moderate
Vliegen et al. 2005[194]	Yes	Yes	Yes	Yes	Yes	Yes	Yes	NR	NR	Yes	Yes	Yes	Yes	Yes	NR	Low
Kim et al. 2004[196]	Yes	Yes	Yes	Yes	Yes	Yes	Yes	NR	NR	Yes	Yes	Yes	Yes	Yes	Yes	Low
Okizuka et al. 1996[195]	Yes	NR	NR	Yes	Yes	No	Yes	NR	NR	Yes	Yes	Yes	Yes	Yes	NR	Moderate

www.ingramcontent.com/pod-product-compliance
Lightning Source LLC
Chambersburg PA
CBHW081721170526
45167CB00009B/3654